Praise for *Laugh to De*

"I never knew Martin Welsh, but I feel as though I did, thanks to this wise, honest, inspiring, and very funny—that's right, funny—book about his struggle with ALS. He was a remarkable man and a gifted writer. And I'm not just saying that because he used my columns as a cure for constipation."

—Dave Barry
Humor columnist, *Miami Herald*

"*Laugh to Death* is not just about dying, it's about living. This book empowers those who feel powerless and cuts to the core of the matter: our mutual mortality. Facing death gave Dr. Martin Welsh a clarity that few ever grasp, allowing us to reap the benefits of his wisdom, insight, and humor."

—Mike Bernhagen and Terry Kaldhusdal
Co-producers, *Consider the Conversation*

"Let me make it easy for you—buy this book! *Laugh to Death* is at times as wry and witty as a *Saturday Night Live* episode, and ripe with the gentle irony of a man who gets what is important in life and makes sure we don't miss the point."

—Jeremy Nobel, M.D.
Faculty, Harvard Medical School
President, Foundation for Art & Healing

"*Laugh to Death* is the perfect title to describe author Dr. Martin Welsh, who never let his ALS diagnosis get the better of him. Marty found humor and joy in every situation as his disease progressed. His unique perspective as doctor becoming patient makes this a perfect book for anyone dealing with a terminal diagnosis, whether patient, caregiver, or medical provider."

—Catherine Lomen-Hoerth, M.D., Ph.D.
Director, ALS Center at UCSF
Professor of Clinical Neurology

Laugh to Death

My Rx for Dying Well with ALS

MARTIN F. WELSH, M.D.

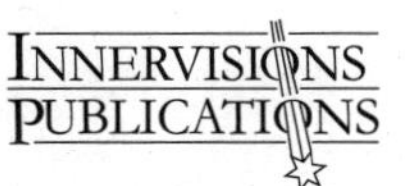

Coloma, California

Published by: Innervisions Publications
PO Box 213
Coloma, CA 95613
intuitivegg@yahoo.com
Editors: Diana Sherer, Write My Wrongs
Cover design: Janice St. Marie
Production: Gina Giacomini
Front and back cover photo credit: Maureen Gill

First Edition

Publisher's Cataloging-in-Publication Data
provided by Five Rainbows Cataloging Services

Names: Welsh, Martin F., author.
Title: Laugh to death : my Rx for dying well with ALS/Martin F. Welsh, M.D.
Description: Coloma, CA : Innervisions, 2018.
Identifiers: LCCN 2018940008|ISBN 978-0-9669427-4-3 (pbk.)|ISBN 978-0-9669427-5-0 (ebook)
Subjects: LCSH: Amyotrophic lateral sclerosis--Patients--Biography. | Death--Psychological aspects. |
Terminally ill--Conduct of life. | Attitude(Psychology) | Autobiography. | BISAC: BIOGRAPHY & AUTOBIOGRAPHY / Personal Memoirs. | BIOGRAPHY & AUTOBIOGRAPHY / Medical. | SOCIAL SCIENCE / Death & Dying.
Classification: LCC RC406.A24 W457 2018 (print) | LCC RC406.A24 (ebook)|DDC 362.1968/390092--dc23.

1 3 5 7 9 10 8 6 4 2

Printed in Canada

To my wife, Maureen Elizabeth Gill,
and the two remarkably admirable young adults I helped raise,
Carey Arlene Welsh and Kevin Callaghan Welsh

ACKNOWLEDGMENTS

~

There are too many people to thank for helping with this book. Inevitably, I'll leave someone out, so to begin with I would like to thank [insert your name here]. So you know who you are, and I've obviously forgotten. After all, I'm demented.

First and foremost, I have to thank my wife Maureen Gill. She edited almost everything before anyone else saw it. On top of that, she coordinated the circus our lives became over the ensuing years. I couldn't have written this book (or lived this long) without her.

I never set out to write a book. I briefly considered writing one when I first diagnosed myself with ALS, so I approached the professional writer in the family, my sister Melinda. I owe her. She recommended a couple of books about the craft, which I read at night in bed. I especially remember Anne Lamott's *Bird by Bird*. I admired her dedication with keeping a journal and writing two hours a day. As for me, yuck! Too much work and commitment. I decided to play golf and travel instead. Then I lived so damn long, and lost the ability to do so much, that writing became the only thing to do. Now, I'm racing the clock to finish this turkey since my arms get very tired of hunt-and-peck typing.

I'd like to thank a second-grade classmate (I think it was James Domenico) who found a way to make us all laugh, wisecracking about anything. I thought, "Being funny—now that's a cool thing." So I've been consciously working at it for forty-eight years, an effort that, hopefully, made you buy this book.

Numerous people have helped me edit this pile of horseshit besides Maureen. Among them were my sister Melinda Welsh and good friend Stacey Leung-Crawford, both professional writers and editors, who assisted with my "shitty first draft." Their comments were insightful and of great help.

My thanks to Sue Horton and her colleagues at the *Los Angeles Times* for helping me edit and publish my essay titled "100 Things Leading to a Single Choice" in the July 2009 issue. This piece got the ball of possibility rolling.

I am also grateful to my good friend Vickie Sugich for taking on the mind-numbing tasks of converting and assembling the first-draft manuscript from computer to paper.

I wish to thank countless comedians and humorists through the years who have shown me the path of looking at things with eyes crossed and logical brain disengaged. A couple of recent examples include writer Dave Barry and comedian Craig Ferguson. Imitation truly is the most sincere form of flattery.

In addition, I wish to thank the people who have kept me alive and functioning longer than I expected: Cathy Lomen-Hoerth, M.D., and her ALS team at University of California, San Francisco; my friend, partner, and family doctor Mark Kal, M.D.; and Mary Walden and the folks who introduced me to the benefits of alternative mental healthcare measures.

I would be remiss not to mention my wonderful legion of caregivers—among them, Bonita Wilson, the first to see me buck naked in a nonsexual situation and make me feel okay with it; Maria Perez; Jessica Pingree; Leah Turner; Tarah Coombs; and Tammy Curbello. They kept me laughing and upbeat in addition to tending to my advancing physical needs.

I owe a great deal to Maureen's parents, Allen and Pat Gill, for showing me how to face the end of life with grace, dignity, and humor. I also want to thank my siblings—Katie, Melinda, Tony, Greg, and David—and their families; my children, Carey and Kevin; my in-laws, who encouraged me throughout by keeping me connected, laughing, and centered on the important things in life. Many of my former patients have kept in touch and lifted my spirits, especially Dan Quayle (not the former VP!), who came to my house again and again over the years, doing the fix-it tasks for me.

My editor, publisher, and agent also deserve special mention, but as of this writing, I have no bloody idea who they may be. You are either brilliant for choosing to publish this work or complete idiots for believing in me.

Lastly, I want to thank the National ALS Association, especially the Sacramento chapter, for the work they do, always with a smile and upbeat attitude in the face of this disaster that is ALS. Like the musicians who kept playing on the *Titanic's* deck as it sank, they bring comfort to those who face certain death before their time. They are angels. Thank you, and may a cure be found soon.

CONTENTS

~

Laugh to Death

FOREWORD

~

My husband Martin, "Marty," Welsh, died on October 28, 2010, at home surrounded by his loving family. *Laugh to Death,* a collection of Marty's writings and short stories, is an enlightening, inspiring, and sometimes hilarious glimpse into the mind and life of a brilliant doctor, loving husband, father, and brother who died much too early, at fifty-six, from Lou Gehrig's disease, ALS.

Initially, after his diagnosis, Marty started writing "ALS Update" emails to keep family and friends informed of his condition. Everyone enjoyed his emails so much, that he decided to start writing funny short stories about his experiences. Both eventually led to the creation of *Laugh to Death*. Marty worked on this book project until the week before his death. For the introduction he chose the following story from the Taoist tradition, "Parable of a Chinese Farmer," a tale that resonated with him greatly as he faced his fate with ALS. I believe he wanted to share the lessons it held with all of us: take life as it comes, the good and the bad; trust what the future holds; and, most importantly, appreciate each day. These are the guidelines Marty tried his best to practice during the six years he lived with ALS.

Parable of a Chinese Farmer

A long, long time ago there lived a farmer whose wife had died. He had a small piece of land he worked with the help of his teenage son and one horse, named Jack, to pull the plough. He barely managed to make a living for the two of them and take care of the horse.

One night Jack escaped and ran off. The neighbor came by and said, "That's bad! Now you've lost your only horse!"

But the farmer said, "Well, you never know."

The next day Jack returned, leading a mare with him into the corral. The neighbor came by and said, "That's good! Now you have two horses!"

But the farmer said, "Well, you never know."

The next day the teenage son thought he'd try to ride the mare, but she was wild and bucked him, causing the boy to fall hard and break his leg. He would be on crutches for months. The neighbor came by and said, "That's bad!"

But the farmer said, "Well, you never know."

The next day the army came marching through town, conscripting all the young men to go off and fight a war. They didn't want the farmer's son since he had a broken leg. The neighbor came by and said, "That's good!"

But the farmer said, "Well, you never know."

—Maureen Gill

PREFACE

~

This book is about attitude.

We aging boomers and our loved ones already face, or soon will, a variety of unwanted detours on our path of an idealized middle and older age. Whether it's heart disease, arthritis, emphysema, cancer, or ALS, something is going to come along to upset your apple cart, or maybe it already has. Psychologically and emotionally, you have a choice of how to deal with these things. I'm not kidding—after the initial shock, you really do have a choice.

But before I get into that, I have to cover the obvious—it's a bit odd writing this preface for a book that might be published (if ever) after I'm dead. How will I do a book signing tour? Maybe they could put my ashes in an urn or an old mayonnaise jar on the table at Barnes and Noble; maybe I'll be floating around as a ghost, or in hell, or maybe heaven, or as a cow in India, or enjoying the forty virgins (I hope they're not nuns).

More importantly, how do you write a funny, enjoyable book about disability, gradually becoming paralyzed, and facing certain death in your fifties? You have to be demented ☑, a bit insane ☑, and have time on your hands ☑. Bingo!

This is *not* meant to be another book about one person's struggles with ALS (a.k.a., Lou Gehrig's disease). ALS is certainly the backdrop of this book, although I intend to go beyond that. Let me make it perfectly clear that it's not going to be your typical, inspirational, tragedy-befell-me-but-I-overcame-it book.

That said, here is the background you need to know about ALS. It's a progressive neurological illness that slowly paralyzes you, muscle by muscle until you die. There is no cure and none in sight. The average life expectancy is three to five years. All the while, you remain fully awake, alert, and aware of what is happening. Most people with ALS die because of respiratory failure (in other words, they can't breathe). ALS happens worldwide and knows no boundaries, no racial or socioeconomic status. It's simply a bad roll of the dice.

Only about 30,000 people in the United States have ALS and each year, 5,600 new cases are diagnosed, replacing those of us who die off. There is only one FDA-approved drug for this illness called Rilutek. This drug may slow it down, although studies have demonstrated a delay time of only two months if you're lucky enough to tolerate the side effects—and if you even think it's worthwhile.

There is some research happening on stem cells, and everyone is excited about them, but those prospects are years or decades away at best. I'll be long gone by then. So, let's run through the attitude options, if or when you get some bad news. The first thing that happens is you feel depressed and sad which can lead to an attitude of self-pity. It's natural, it's normal, and I've been in that place many days in the last few years. But it serves no useful purpose in the long run, does it? Strike one. And so, I sought alternatives.

You could seek solace in faith or religion, and many do. It can be a wonderful source of psychological, and sometimes even physical, comfort. I was raised Catholic but spent my adult life as an agnostic. Lately, a few things have made me realize the power of looking outside my personal woes and upwards, although I have not suddenly become religious again. So, I'm not a spiritual writer as a means of comfort, and it usually doesn't take the pain away, allow me to talk, or make my legs move again. Strike two, at least for me.

I'm angry sometimes, as I have been all my life. But when I let my anger out, usually with vitriol and inappropriate force, I always regret the consequences. I'm occasionally just plain moody and miserable to be around (why only *occasionally* is beyond my comprehension), but thankfully that seems to pass. Scratch that as a helpful option. I can't blame anyone or anything (like toxic exposure) for ALS, but then again, what if I could? Would I end up wasting my precious little time pursuing lawsuits or chasing unproven cures? Strike three.

So I chose insanity as my goal, or as some kindly euphemize it, humor, of course. It works best for me. It hides my anger, my sadness, and self-pity—even from me! It's also socially acceptable. It makes people want to be around and care for me. It was a no-brainer.

Plus, it was easy for me because all my life, I have always had a good, although warped, sense of humor. But seriously, following my own "ALS Rules" (found in Chapter Ten) has made it easier to deal with this truckload of horse manure that was dumped on me in the prime of my life. Rule 7 is about laughing and keeping others laughing and has helped me so far—I hope it helps a few people by showing them a different way to cope with these speed bumps in life.

And I don't claim to be the first to use this approach. For example, I was privileged to hear Norman Cousins, the journalist, author, and peace advocate, speak at UCLA Medical School in 1977. He shared how he laughed his way out of a painful and supposedly terminal illness. Unfortunately, I don't think I'll have his success. And there have been many others as well, including some with ALS.

As my physical abilities gradually vanished and also having the personality I do, I felt a need to stay busy as time passed. I began writing "ALS Update" emails to keep distant family and friends up to speed with the latest news. At first, it was only some twenty-odd people, but now, as of July 2010, I must be sending out well over a hundred copies each time.

Then, some interesting and funny things happened along the way, so I started writing stories about them. People told me I was a decent writer and that I ought to make a book out of the whole mess. If you're reading this, then they were right.

I hope you bought this book because you heard it was quite entertaining, or it made you laugh when you thought you should feel guilty for not crying, or it helps you change how you deal with disability and death, or because—best scenario—Oprah recommended it.

One sad part for me is that I won't be able to write my second book which would be entitled *Before the Truckload of Lemons Arrived.*

A lot of funny stuff has happened to me in my life, and only some of you have heard the stories. I'm relying on you to share them with others and laugh when you think of me. Even if you're laughing at me and not with me, it's okay. Humor is the most wonderful attribute we humans have.

If you are laughing *at* me, just watch out for the rake on the stairs next time you go down into the creepy basement. I may just choose the ghost option.

One

I Diagnose Myself, and No One Believes Me

~

Ever since I was a child, I wanted to be a doctor. I was the oldest of six children—there were seven next door and another handful up and down the block. I was somehow drawn into becoming the neighborhood medic. My mother died when I was twelve years old, and my dad worked long hours to support us; consequently, whenever my brothers, sisters, or a neighbor kid got a scrape or bruise, they came to me. I remember enjoying bandaging them up after making them cry. I used a lot of tincture of Merthiolate—remember that stuff? It stings, and Bactine was for sissies! But they kept coming to me. Then there was the influence of the *Marcus Welby, M.D.* show on TV. I won't tell you about the trouble I got myself into when I found a bunch of insulin syringes and needles in the gutter one day. You can just imagine.

Lucky enough to inherit the intelligence required, I was focused and persistent enough to achieve my goal. I got my M.D. from UCLA in 1980. I spent three more years becoming board certified in family practice. I moved to a small town in the Northern California Sierra foothills to work and raise a family. It was a script I had written when I was seven.

I had a good career going in Placerville with lots of patients who loved me—many became good friends as well. My two kids were "A" students, and I managed to make enough free time to satisfy my addiction to playing sports: basketball, tennis, water-skiing, long-distance running, and golf. Appointed chief of staff at the local hospital in 1990, I've been a respected member of the community, blah, blah, blah.

Fast forward.

There's a common saying among the medical community about family practice, and it's true: good family practice is the first ten minutes of every specialty. In other words, a family practice doctor studies all the medical specialties and knows a little about each one. I found this to be especially true in the following incident. In May 2004, I conducted a full neurological exam on a patient (I've since completely blanked on who it was or why). Depending on the patient's symptoms, I did this exam anywhere from once a week to once a month. Anyway, part of it calls for *rapid, alternating movements.* I face the patient and start by tapping my thumb and index finger rapidly together. As I demonstrated this movement on my left hand, he mimicked with his right. Then, when I did the same on my right hand, I noticed my movements were definitely slower than my left. The patient didn't notice, but I was puzzled as I finished the exam.

The rest of that day as I sat at my desk, I periodically rechecked myself, and it stayed the same. Later on, I collared Mark Kal, my friend, partner, and a family practice doctor, and said, "Hey Mark, look at this." He asked if I had any wrist pain. I didn't, so he checked me for cogwheel rigidity, a sign of Parkinson's disease. He then looked at me and said, "I want you to go see Rajiv" (Dr. Rajiv Pathak, our local neurologist). Mark got right on the phone, and, two days later, there I was in Rajiv's office.

Rajiv found the same thing, and also noticed that my reflexes were stronger in my right arm than the left. Abnormal, we both knew. Rajiv did a quick test for carpal tunnel syndrome which we both knew would be negative. He then ordered a battery of blood tests and set me up for an MRI of my brain and cervical spinal cord. After all, even with no neck pain, it was possible I had a disc pinching a nerve. The blood tests, including the first of several repeats for HIV and Lyme disease, all came back normal, and I knew this as I sat awaiting my MRI.

I don't claim to be a brilliant diagnostician, but I realized it was down to one of four things: a small stroke, a brain tumor, multiple sclerosis, or ALS. I knew the first three would show up on the MRI. So I calmly had the scan, and my radiologist friend and colleague of twenty-three years called me into the reading room to go over the pictures.

As I walked in the room, he said the words I've never forgotten: "Good news, Marty. Your scans are normal." It was the end of the day on May 28, 2004, and I knew I had ALS. No doubt in my mind. I thanked him—saying nothing, of course—walked to my car, and drove home. Understandably, I was on autopilot and emotionally numb.

When I got home, I told my wife Maureen the results and what I thought. She wouldn't or couldn't believe it. Same with Mark. So, I told no one else. I carried on with business as usual.

In July 2004, Rajiv finally convinced me to see an ALS specialist in San Francisco. He was suspicious but didn't offer a definitive diagnosis. He wanted to see me again in three months. What I remember of that summer was that I suffered psychologically because I knew I had it, but neither Mark, Rajiv, nor my wife believed me. I just couldn't have ALS—it must be something different. Of course, the underlying truth was they didn't want me to have it.

Over the course of three days in October, we had the follow-up visit in San Francisco and got a second opinion from another ALS specialist. They both confirmed what I had known all summer. Only then did Maureen break down and cry. Then the planning started: how and when to tell everyone, how to plan when to retire, what to do with the rest of my life. Enough of that for now—let's fast forward again.

Let me tell you a secret—I will die at the end. But, so what? To the best of my knowledge, every human who has ever been born has died. Whether that happens at five minutes, five years, fifty-five, or ninety-five, it's almost always a sad event—with a few exceptions (Adolph Hitler comes to mind). I may come off as cruel-minded and heartless here, but I'm the one who's dying. So, to grossly misuse the words of a song by the Eagles, "Get Over It."

So began my journey and discovery of the importance of attitude.

TWO

I Encounter a Brief Interruption

~

An interesting thing happened in September 2004, less than four months after I discovered I was going to die (and statistically soon) from ALS. One afternoon at work while using the toilet in the clinic, there was blood in my urine. Painless. Once. It quickly vanished and never returned.

I made the mistake of telling Mark, my doctor and good friend, who set me up for a CAT scan of my kidneys. This test turned out normal, so he suggested I go to the urologist for a cystoscopy. For some reason, he didn't trust me and my minor symptoms anymore.

Cystoscopy is a delightful procedure where they stick a flexible fiber-optic tube up your pecker and take a look inside your bladder. I knew I had to have this, it was no big deal and done in the office. But, being a typical male, I was thrilled, of course, not to mention what my pecker thought. I made my appointment for the end of the week.

On the appointed day, I finished work early, did my paperwork, walked across the parking lot to the urologist's office, was led into the procedure room, dropped my pants and waited. A cute, young medical assistant came in, had me lie down on the power table and proceeded to clean off my business with an antiseptic solution. I thought she might be nervous knowing I was an M.D., so I tried to make small talk and asked, "How long have you been working for Dr. Desai?"

"I'm just in training," she replied, and proceeded to squirt a tube of local anesthetic up my urethra and put a hose clamp on my weenie to keep it there. "Dr. Desai will be here in a minute."

"This is going well so far," I thought.

Desai walked in and quickly got to it. We were talking shop when all of a sudden, he said, "Marty! You've got a bladder tumor! What are you doing with a bladder tumor?" (Medical note: *All* bladder tumors are, by default, cancerous.) I think I said that I had no idea, but I was a bit nonplussed. Only four months ago, I'd discovered I had an incurable, fatal disease. What happened to the nonsmoking, fit athlete who preached to his patients the benefits of a healthy lifestyle, day in and day out?

Then, he said, "Do you want to see it?" So, get the visual here: I'm lying flat on my back, naked from the waist down, having just exposed my privates to a high school girl, and he has this two-foot-long black hose inserted up my schnauzer with an eyepiece attached.

I said, "I don't think I can."

And he said, "Sure you can!" Then, he hit the button in front of me. I'm looking at my wiener with a black hose coming out of it, and he hands me the eyepiece. I swear, I'm not making this up.

So, I got a peek at my cancer. It looked innocent enough—like a sea anemone on a short stalk, waving its fingers in the current of water. But there it was, as big as a golf ball.

I left his office, thinking to myself, "What the hell is happening to me?" In the car on the drive home, while making the left turn to get on the freeway, a guy nearly t-boned me doing over forty mph and running a red light! I slammed on the brakes, and he swerved wildly to avoid hitting me. I was numb all the way home, and I got into the scotch pretty good that night. Don't remember much else.

To make quick work of the rest, I had surgery to remove the tumor and told the surgeon and anesthesiologist, in confidence, that I had early ALS which they needed to know. The surgery went well. It turned out to be the lowest grade cancer and had not gone into the stalk yet. I didn't need chemotherapy and was most likely cured.

Nevertheless, I had cancer for crying out loud! One of Mark's patients who was about my age had just recently died miserably from bladder cancer. I was starting to feel a little paranoid, but I had more pressing issues to resolve, so I decided to put the bladder cancer on my mental back burner.

THREE

Time's Fun When You're Having Flies

~

It's February 2005, and I'm eight months past my first symptoms. Change is moving at a glacial pace. My right hand moves slowly, I can't play the guitar as well as I used to (I wasn't great to start with), and my arm feels a bit funny some days more than others. It's like trying to watch the grass grow—so on most days, I don't pay attention. On Mondays, the alarm goes off at six; I get up, go to work, and do it again Tuesday, etc. Eventually, I realize another week has gone by. I am the same and not dead yet.

I've been on Rilutek, the one and only Rx for ALS, for a month now with no side effects. It sometimes causes liver problems, so I'm having blood tests, and the first set turned out normal. I'm back to drinking scotch before the bottle of wine with dinner every day.

I'm taking a bunch of pills now, though—a real change for nature boy. Besides a baby aspirin (because I turned fifty), I now take a multivitamin, 1000mg C, 400mg E, fish oil, flax oil, and the Rilutek twice a day. I feel like my eighty-year-old patients with their bags of pills! I've even resorted to one of those weekly pill container jobs! *That's* depressing.

Never much of a gym person, my back now bothers me when I try to run, so I'm doing the elliptical and treadmill thing. And a few weeks ago, I got started on routinely hitting the weight room machines, thinking I needed to make the most of what's still working as time passes. I notice a very slight difference in what my right arm can do, but it's still very subtle, and only I can tell the difference because no one is testing me.

And because it's winter up here, there's not as much opportunity to golf, but I was at the range last Sunday, and nothing had changed. My game is not miraculously better—all the same old problems. Damn! But it got me thinking that I should do something insane. So yesterday—in a driving rainstorm—I went over to a local country club and wrote a check. We've now officially left the public course ranks and joined the elitist, chauvinistic, good-old-boy network of private golf club members. I had to go to the thrift store to get plaid pants and ugly shirts, but it's in the club bylaws to dress like Rodney Dangerfield in *Caddyshack.* Now I have to stay good with the arm despite the f**king ALS.

As for the bladder cancer, I just yesterday had my first three-month follow-up cystoscopy to see if it was still dead/missing/not there anymore. I told the urologist I didn't want any surprises this time when he looked in there, and it was okay—all clear. I walked back across the parking lot and finished up the day's paperwork. F**k bladder cancer, too, while I'm at it.

Now, it's May 2005, one year since I learned I had ALS and was going to die prematurely. It's definitely been an interesting year, emotionally and psychologically. Between this and the bladder cancer, I've had a rude splash of ice water thrown on me. How the hell did I get these things? All my professional and personal life, I have lived and preached a healthy lifestyle for a long and prosperous existence. Now, I get hit by these two stray bullets? But somehow, I haven't gotten into a funk about it. Don't ask me why, because I don't know. Now, I look at it as having my cake and eating it, too—I have this intense appreciation for life, and almost every day is special. Plus, I'm not going away in a big hurry. You should all be jealous!

To all external appearances, nothing is different. No one can tell or knows about my disability unless we tell them. My right hand is a little weaker—my grip strength went from 140 to 92 over the past year. In general, my right arm is a little weaker, but no one seems to notice except me. A year ago, I didn't observe any slowness or difficulty writing. I do now.

Just a year ago, I could play the guitar; I'd just lose the pick in my fingers (I can still hear my brothers laughing). Now, I can't strum rhythmically. A year ago, I could dribble a basketball and shoot it, which I discovered a month ago is something else that is now gone. It requires a quick wrist flick, and I don't do "quick" anymore. Thankfully, swinging a golf club is a two-handed affair, so my left helps my right, and I'm still the same mediocre golfer I was previously.

I've made some adjustments at work to compensate, although I continue at it full-time and have no imminent plans to slow down or quit. That will probably change if and when my right arm goes entirely south. With the benefit of a year's time to gauge the pace of this thing, I'd guess my schedule will change in the next year.

I just had the follow-up MRI scans and a neurology visit, and there's no change of diagnosis. The only definite findings are still limited to my right arm. The local neurologist maintains his cautious skepticism about the diagnosis because although I have weakness, slowness, and hyper reflexes, I don't have the muscle atrophy or fasciculations (brief, spontaneous contractions) in my right hand or arm that usually go with ALS. He wonders if I have this related thing called PLS (primary lateral sclerosis) that is even rarer than ALS, but I'm not that typical for it. He's still in denial. What are friends for, anyway? They hope for the best for you.

I started my weekend off playing golf with a patient of mine who is eighty-nine years old but refuses to act his age. He used to play professional baseball—I love people like that, of course. We teed off at 6:30 a.m., walked the course, and finished the eighteen holes in three hours (which, for you non-golfers, is very fast). And yes—he beat me. A good way to start the day, and what a great example he is!

I occasionally fear, and I do know that the honeymoon won't last. I have dark moments when I think about the likely future, but I snap out of it pretty quickly because what's the point?

Last night, I asked Maureen if she thought I was crazy because I'm feeling so happy and fortunate right now. Because I have this diagnosis, I'm so appreciative of every little thing, the beautiful world around me; every moment of every day; I pity those of you who don't have it. Well, not really. I think you know what I mean. At this point, I consider myself a truly lucky man. So, I'm on to year two of living with this. I doubt it will be as good physically as year one, but you never know.

FOUR

No Surprises and Some Very Good News

~

Maureen and I went to the ALS Center at UCSF in November 2005, since it was time for my routine checkup. We had a three-hour visit and left once again feeling very gratified and confident with their staff and services there.

We heard from Dr. Cathy Lomen-Hoerth that there is more recent data from Europe that the Rilutek drug I'm taking does, indeed, effectively slow down ALS more when started early. This data confirmed the last year's preliminary thoughts, so I'm glad I started it back in January. We talked for a while, then Dr. Cathy examined me and did an EMG testing (an electromyogram tests the electrical activity of muscles).

Over the last year, my right arm has slowly worsened, which is no surprise to anyone. Starting last May, I was pretty sure my right leg was involved, and the EMG showed that. I suspected that my tongue was also showing signs, and Dr. Cathy confirmed that very early findings were also there. So when I sound like I'm drunk at ten in the morning, I'm *not!*

The really good news is my breathing is completely okay so far, as measured by pulmonary function and EMG testing of muscles in my upper back. In summary, Dr. Cathy said that the changes she sees in me after one year are what she usually observes in the first two to three months. So, it's slow, slow, slow. We suspect this is because my case is slow anyway, and the Rilutek makes it even more delayed.

I asked her what she thought of my expectation that working would be feasible (a slower pace and some accommodation) through next spring or summer, and she concurred this seemed about right. So, retirement looms!

On a side note, the San Francisco Bay area is quite pleasant in the fall. We had a nice lunch in Sausalito on the way down and a great dinner at Kuleto's near Union Square before we came home. It turned out to be a good day. We are feeling okay about things at this point, but once again, we need to start rolling on some changes—making some time for my physical fitness/maintenance, notifying my patients, etc.

We both appreciate all the concern and thoughts and prayers sent our way. They help a lot. We're doing fine, so far.

FIVE

Okay, Okay, I'll Take the Pill

~

It's 2006, and I thought it would be romantic to spend Valentine's Day with my wife, sitting in an exam room at the ALS Clinic at UCSF. She swooned with delight. We did stay two nights at the Donatello Hotel and had a great dinner the night before at the Farallon Seafood Restaurant, so it turned out okay. No divorce papers in the mail.

Anyway, this was my first team clinic visit where you arrive at ten in the morning and stay in the same room until five. Meanwhile, a parade of people come by, and each gets a piece of you for thirty minutes: respiratory therapy, physical therapy, occupational therapy, speech and swallow therapy, a social worker, a dietician, a shrink (no kidding!), a representative from the ALS Association, someone from MDA (Muscular Dystrophy Association) ALS division, a wheelchair specialist, the clinic nurse manager (who is brilliant and very capable), then the doctor. Whew! I guess I'm one of Jerry's Kids now!

They are all very familiar with the vagaries of ALS, doing this team thing weekly, monitoring the 300-odd patients followed there. They were all very helpful, and we had a low-key visit since I think I'm one of their least impaired patients at this point. The occupational therapy woman is Irish. She was quite impressed when I told her I recently climbed Croagh Patrick Mountain, in County Mayo, Ireland. It's forty-five degrees or steeper in some places with no switchbacks on loose rock. I did this last June with a bad arm (using a cane) and symptoms starting in my right leg. You'd have to see it and climb it to understand.

At this point, nothing has dramatically changed since I saw them in November 2005, except that the muscles in my right arm and leg are decidedly more spastic and tense. Dr. Cathy had recommended a muscle relaxer medicine back then, but I was a little reluctant since I was a bit worried about the possible side effects of sedation and I thought my gym program, massages, and other alternative stuff might do the trick. Well, no cigar. She also pointed out that my walking and writing might improve with the medication. So, I'm going to take Baclofen three times daily along with my twice daily Rilutek and all the vitamins/ supplements. Cripes! I'm like all my patients over the years who have said, "I could open my own pharmacy with all the stuff I take!"

My walking and balance are a little gimpier, and my speech is thick at times. Everything is worse when I'm cold or tired, but these aren't very noticeable unless you look closely, which most people don't, of course. That's why many of my patients were shocked by the letter I sent out in December, telling them of my ALS and announcing my limited schedule and availability. I've received wonderful responses from them as you can imagine. When they see me, most say, "But you *look* so good and healthy!" That will probably start to change within a year, but for now, it's nice to be without a cane or a brace on my ankle.

I get to drop the other shoe on them shortly with the official letter: "I am retiring as of May 1, 2007." General fatigue and the use of my right hand are the limiting factors that are going to drive me out. I'm grateful I was able to keep pursuing my life's passion for nearly two years after the symptoms started, and no one except me knew what I had.

Maureen and I aren't sitting around waiting for May. We're busy already! I took a week off in February, and we flew to Arizona for a visit to Sedona and the Grand Canyon. I was in Mexico again last weekend for my fourth trip with the Flying Samaritans.

Tomorrow, we head to Yosemite for a quick visit (I've never been there in the snow) and to participate in a close friend's birthday party. I'll take one more week of vacation in March. We'll go back to the Southwest to see my cousin Brian at his oasis date farm, China Ranch. We'll also go through Death Valley (where my mother was born), Bryce Canyon, and Zion National Park. After that, there are only four more weeks, and I'm done!

It's hard to imagine retiring and how this will feel day after day. I start out the first week at Bodega Bay, which was part of my overall timing plan. It has always been a peaceful place for reflection and deep thought for me—not to mention good food, even better wine, and golf! That's right, sports fans—I'm officially on disability, retired, and playing golf. How's that for a paradox? I'm expecting private investigators from the disability company lurking with cameras in the bushes. I'm going to enjoy it while it lasts.

The rest of the year is filling up with my son Kevin's wedding, spending more time with my kids and siblings, and planning vacations. We're thinking about Connecticut, Wisconsin, maybe Montana, and an autumn trip up the coast to Washington and Oregon. I've never done the Shakespeare Festival in Ashland. I'm going to have trouble squeezing in golf days *after* I retire! Then there are ocean cruise opportunities popping up on the radar!

So yes, be jealous of the guy with ALS, at least for now. I caught sight of a few of the other patients at UCSF this week. They were in wheelchairs and having trouble talking. But denial is a great tool for all of us right now. We continue to make good and helpful use of it while we can.

SIX

Wednesday

~

Allow me to tell you about last Wednesday.

Maureen and I awoke in Sedona, Arizona, halfway through our five-day vacation to the Southwest. I had scheduled the week off to visit Mexico with some friends, but when the trip canceled, we retooled our vacation to go to Sedona and the Grand Canyon—places I had never been and was drawn to see. Not the least reason was the reported spiritual nature of Sedona which, as some of you know, is an area of interest to me lately, what with all that's happening in our lives.

We awoke sans alarm clock, a nice break from the routine, and had some breakfast at the motel. We had driven around the area and gone on a hike the day before. Maureen was especially interested in one more stop before we headed north to the big ditch in the ground.

Oak Creek and its tributaries run through the area, and there is a park at a place called Red Rock Crossing which is in the shadow of a stunning piece of geology called Cathedral Rock. It's a several-hundred-foot-high formation carved out by erosion. And it is, well, red, and standing alone like a cathedral. Cathedral Rock is one of the supposed vortex sites in the Sedona area where multiple dimensions supposedly exist beyond the four we experience daily. So, when in Rome, do as the Romans, right?

We parked and were just about the only people there early on a cold February morning. It hadn't rained or snowed for weeks, but the creek was still flowing. It was quite peaceful and beautiful walking around on the trail. The water bubbled, some birds flew about, there was a hawk high in a tree—you get the picture. Convinced there was indeed a crossing, Maureen found it downstream a bit. It was a curving chain of flat stones laid out above the waterline, perfect for crossing the thirty-foot-wide stream that was three feet deep in places and flowing briskly.

I had been having some intermittent dizziness of late. I thought it was partly due to an imbalance in my leg strength, but it was there sometimes even when I sat. Of course, I awoke that morning with this unwelcome guest and was still wobbling a bit as we strolled along the creek. You can see where I'm going with this.

We have a great picture of the stone crossing from the near side of the river. Maureen said, "This looks pretty easy," as she scampered across like those bugs that walk on water.

I thought to myself, "Is she trying to kill me?" So I stood there, looking at the stones, looking in my heart and hearing my brain say, "This may not be a good idea today." It was a classic battle between brains and guts, circa sixth grade. "Hey guys, watch this!" Then, I started out across the river on the stones.

I apologize here because I'm going to disappoint. But diversion is a classic trick in entertainment. I realized five stones into the journey that this was like making a free throw in basketball or a short putt to win a golf match. I had to have supreme confidence knowing that I was going to make it across. I thought about something else while I let my legs do the job. God help me, I started singing a song to myself, and before I knew it, I'd made it across, completely dry. Lesson learned again.

We sat on a nearby rock, looked up at Cathedral Rock, then had a good, if brief, meditation session. I'm doing more of that lately and getting a bit better at it. I finally had a color breakthrough last week, but that's another story. Crossing back was now a piece of cake, and we started our meandering journey out of Sedona.

Sedona is a mecca for artists, with a wide variety of art to be seen, including a lot of Native American (mostly Navaho) art. Our last stop was a most interesting visit to the Goldenstein Art Gallery. We met an artist named Sherab who does paintings and sculptures of Buddha. The sculptures go for about $50,000 (Nicholas Cage has one). The prints are a bargain at $1,000. Sherab had been a Buddhist nun for twelve years and had a very engaging and powerful personality. Both the art and artists made a big impression on us. And so we left Sedona.

Driving north, we climbed up the Colorado Plateau into Flagstaff. It's a quaint little town on old Route 66 where freight trains run through day and night (we know because we heard them all night long when we stayed there on the way home). Anyway, we didn't stop, but proceeded to the Grand Canyon's South Rim entrance and straight to Mather Point, the first place you can park and see the thing. It was an hour before sunset. We took a picture. Everybody takes a photo, showing it to people while saying, "It was much, much grander than this!" It is jaw-dropping spectacular, immense beyond words, one of the wonders of the planet, whatever. Just see it for yourself, will you please?

We had booked a room at El Tovar, a hundred-plus-year-old historic hotel right on the rim. I mean don't wander drunk out the door at night, or you might fall over the railing. We checked in and asked the bellboy (he was only twenty, so he's a boy to me) about the best place to see the sunset.

Following his directions eastward along the rim trail, we walked twenty-five minutes and were rewarded with a great view. Once the sun had set and the darkness was slowly gathering, Rod Sterling cued *The Twilight Zone* music, and here we go again.

We walked back along the unlit path toward the hotel as the shadows grew and my squint narrowed. Suddenly, Maureen grabbed my arm and cried out, "Look, Marty, what's that?" She was instantly fearful—not a usual response for her—this reaction is interesting later.

What she saw that I missed was a single bighorn ram walking along the path toward us. He was maybe three feet at the shoulder, looked very muscular and healthy with a set of formidable horns. He was walking on the human's asphalt path in the forest, not breaking stride, not paying any attention to us (although he undoubtedly saw us long before we saw him), and on our side of the path, playing chicken with us.

I didn't think he looked mean or aggressive. He was just cruising along while acting very alpha, so we decided we should get out of his way. We got off the path and stood behind a tree as he passed. I could have reached out and touched him. He ignored us, walked on, and disappeared into the darkness. We got back to the hotel, had a good stiff drink in the bar and a nice dinner, then we went to bed.

So, what the heck was that about? We told the bellboy what we'd seen, and he was incredulous. Since we had just come from this spiritual nexus in Sedona, we thought this experience had a deeper meaning or was some kind of omen. It turns out that Native Americans assigned the meaning of bighorn sheep to transitions or new beginnings, according to a reference book I read. I'm no expert, and that was just a single book, but it wouldn't take Einstein to connect those dots. As for my transition, I'm planning on retiring at the end of April.

Before some of you think I've lost it and fallen off my rocker, please be reassured that, at this point, I just find this stuff engaging and fascinating. I'm a scientist by nature and training, and if someone isn't skeptical entering med school, they quickly learn to be. I aced that class, just so you know.

This spirituality, meditation, zero-point field, quantum physics, *What the Bleep* stuff is kind of interesting now and is one of the silver linings I keep talking about as I/we go through this journey with ALS.

So that was Wednesday.

SEVEN

I Need to Retire from Retirement

~

We took a second trip to the Southwest at the end of March 2007, spending time with my cousin Brian at his China Ranch in the desert. We headed to Utah, back to Arizona for the Glen Canyon Dam and Lake Powell, then to Utah again for Zion, and finally, Bryce. All these places were wonderful; although, no more eerie ram sightings.

I worked four final weeks in April, and I had the idea of taking a picture with each of the last month's patients. Word got out, and pretty soon my patients were just dropping by (because of my booked schedule) to be part of the photos taken. I ended up with nearly 200 pictures of my friends smiling with me. That's certainly nowhere near all of them, but it's a good representation. It made quite an album to look through as the years pass.

The staff gave me a terrific going-away party, and the gift was a marvelous scrapbook of everyone. I will cherish it always. Maureen came by that last evening and helped me pack up my office and clean it out since my replacement arrived the next day. As previously arranged, she drove me home as a precaution, although the reality and the emotions of leaving didn't hit for a couple of days.

Maureen helped my medical group plan and orchestrate my official retirement party (a roast) on May 7. It turned out to be a great day. My kids came up for the weekend, and everyone was too nice instead of roasting me as they could have.

These last three months have been a blur of activity: the whole retirement thing, the Bodega Bay week, a three-day golf tournament, the annual Welsh Brothers' reunion, a quick trip to King City and one to

Walnut Creek, my son Kevin's wedding weekend, one last trip with the Flying Samaritans to Mexico, a five-day road trip to Southern California, and—what am I forgetting? Oh yeah, *we moved!*

We had started looking in January and finally found the perfect house one week before I retired. Miserable timing, but there it was. In the midst of all of the above, we've been going through escrow, moving, sorting through boxes, and dealing with contractors for small jobs on both houses. We have been struggling with internet access at the new house and are still trying to get the old place emptied out, fixed up, and on the market.

I need a vacation from my retirement. So, I have recently started to volunteer as a mentor of sorts to some of the new, younger docs in the group. I also want to pop in and visit a few special patients now and then while I can. If nothing else, it'll get me out of Maureen's hair for a while. I pity her now that I'm home every day.

It has been over two years since I first noticed it in my hand and diagnosed myself—not quite a year since I had an *official* confirmation at a clinic visit. My symptoms are slowly progressing, as expected, but the main good news is that there is no new area of involvement—my left arm and leg are okay as best as I can tell. My right leg gives me more trouble than my arm and hand, maybe because more strength is required to walk than to use my arm. I always use a cane now. I tire pretty quickly and need to sit down a lot. I haven't had any bad falls yet, and that's nice. I'm extremely careful because it's a long way down for me! Like all else, walking is sometimes better or worse, but I often think I'll be ready for a wheelchair before a year passes.

My speech is also getting worse, so I sound thick-tongued and drunk at times, even though I'm not (I think those days are gone). I have improved my ambidextrous capabilities, so the hand thing doesn't interfere too much. Depending on the situation, I use either hand now to eat. I even taught myself to use chopsticks with my left hand since I'm too proud to ask for a fork.

My last clinic visit was shorter than before, partly because they didn't send in the shrink. They must sense that we're hopeless and there's no helping us. The only surprising change was that although my breathing force remains at the top of the chart, my lung capacity has dropped off quite a bit. I'm scheduled for an overnight oxygen measuring test this week; they gave me some breathing exercises to do—along with the toy for doing them!

I have my own personal Ambu bag now for breathing exercises. I promptly made light of it, using it as a prop for a video we shot with my brother Greg's kids in Escondido. Another new addition I'll soon have is an AFO which is a brace for my right ankle. My calf muscles are very weak, and this should help me stay upright a little longer. Enough of the *bad* news.

I'm still golfing! No more walking the course, and hills are hard, but I can finish eighteen holes. I use a club as a cane when walking to the ball from my golf cart, and my balance is mostly okay when I swing. I'm adjusting to lost distance, of course, but that's okay. I'm pretty tired by the end of the round, and that's it for the day, but so what?

Interesting things continue to happen—along the lines of that mystical encounter with the ram in February, the visual stuff I see when meditating, and when Mary Walden, my massage therapist and friend, works on me. The hardest to believe is me winning a putting tournament (the field included fifty or so participants) while a group of friends focused and meditated about me. The strangest experience of all was when our friend Diane Bush was doing a Feng Shui consultation at the house. During the session, I saw a variety of colors. I'm sure there are various explanations for all of this, including some insights from friends and my former Roman Catholic beliefs. But at this point, I'm "just observing," as someone put it.

Life goes on, and I'm enjoying every day tremendously. As I've said before, this diagnosis has helped me understand and practice the Zen of being in the moment. Lots of fun things are on the horizon. I have an appointment again at UCSF on October 31! What a sense of humor they have! If it stands, we'll stay the night to experience Halloween in San Francisco.

EIGHT

Chopsticks, Walkers ... and Still Golfing

~

Here's your intrepid reporter giving you news from the front lines after another visit to the ALS Clinic in November 2007. It'll be brief because most of the news was boring.

Let me tell you what a stubborn fool I am. Now when I limp into a Chinese restaurant, I wear a brace on my right ankle and hold a cane with my left hand since my right arm is nearly useless for that. When they serve me, I ask for chopsticks because I'd rather look ridiculous using my left hand than resort to a fork. If I used chopsticks or a fork with my right hand, I'd be flinging noodles onto the next table.

Any activity—the morning routine in the bathroom, showering and shaving, or getting dressed without the brace—wears me out like a heavy workout did in the past. So, I'm going to be seen shortly with a late model, high performance, all the bells and whistles—walker. And a wheelchair is approaching like Secretariat down the home stretch.

The clinic visit itself was interesting because I was smothered with students. There were two students from physical therapy and a third-year medical student. The medical student was very nervous and told me I could correct her on her neurological exam technique. I would've had more fun torturing her, but my wife was there. It was odd for me because for ten years I did teach third-year students from UC Davis.

There were some things she needed to hear (and a bunch I could have made up), but I restrained myself and acted as a good patient, with one exception. Dr. Cathy has been following me for two years now, so I asked her some questions about prognosis—the kind of stuff we doctors never can answer with any level of certainty. She said that I could probably avoid total dependence on a wheelchair for another year. Of course, it'll be a gradual transition. The rest hinges on the breathing part (mostly on the force measurement), so it's hard to say until that starts declining. She thinks I have at least three more years to live, but certainly not ten. That's the good/bad news about a slowly progressive course. I am enjoying this period now, but I don't particularly want an extended period of real dependence ... duh!

So as not to end on a downer note, I'm still playing golf! I have to take it easy the day before and the day after, or I'm whacked. Fortunately, with the leg brace and driving the golf cart as close as possible to my ball, I can still play eighteen holes for the time being. I run out of gas after fourteen holes or so, and I limp home. My handicap is skyrocketing into the stratosphere which still bugs me to no end. I have this delusion that if I play smarter, am conservative with my shot selection, and improve my short game, then I can score better. But it hasn't happened yet. Oh well, I'm still out there for a little while longer.

Oh, and by the way, I had my two-year follow-up check on the bladder cancer yesterday. It's that lovely procedure called cystoscopy—it was my last one because the cancer is gone, gone, gone. It's one less thing to worry about.

NINE

Pebble Beach

~

The only news worth mentioning from my clinic visit in March 2007, is that my breathing is doing very well, indeed. When the ALS started, my baseline measured at 98 percent; it had previously dipped to 94 in February 2006. Last summer, I could only manage 84 percent (a rude shock!), so they started me on some breathing exercises. I hit 92 last week. That probably is part of the reason my stamina has noticeably improved since last fall. My sleep is better, and I cough less.

As of now, I like the stamina improvement because it means my prediction that I'd be in a wheelchair part-time at this stage has proven erroneous. My right leg is definitely weakening, but I walk okay with the AFO leg brace and my cane. Although I'm finding it harder and am a little unsteady, I haven't fallen in nearly a year, so I'm still playing golf! The icing on the cake is—my scores are even a bit better than last fall. By Christmas, my golfing days will be done, so each time out is a blessing.

Speaking of blessings, Mrs. Santa Claus surprised me with a tee time at Pebble Beach on December 30! Maureen and I played a round at the West Coast shrine of golf with her brother David and his best friend Clem (who caddied for him in 2000 when he won the AT&T Pebble Beach amateur title). Needless to say, this is quite a memory to have. Unfortunately, my golf stunk by that time, and Pebble Beach is a very, very hard course. The ocean feasted on my balls. I mean, of course, my golf balls.

Sadly, my speech is still going south, so I sound like a sloppy drunk most of the time. I'm close to requesting a recommendation for some kind of assistive device. I may get one of those computer voice devices and start talking like HAL in the movie, *2001: A Space Odyssey*. Maybe I can program it with different voices, a thick Sean Connery brogue one day, Austin Powers the next, and Antonio Banderas on the weekends.

My right hand is barely changing. I still use the computer mouse, and I haven't modified the double-click speed setting, which seems odd since the ALS started there nearly three years ago.

More and more, I'm a lefty for eating. I noticed the other night that I now reach for a fork or glass with my left hand without even thinking about it. I am transitioning to writing left-handed, especially if it is more than signing my name or writing a couple of words.

I'm pretty sure that it's also started in my left leg, although not much has changed there in six months, so I'm not paying much attention yet. Nothing wrong with the left arm yet, which is a good thing!

I just started participating in a trial through UCSF which involves a very high dose of CoQ10, a supplement you can buy in 100mg tablets. I'm either taking 2,700mg a day—or placebo! We'll see. (It turned out I was on the real thing, and the study showed it had no effect.)

In December, I got a suggestion to formalize some of my ideas that had helped me cope, so I came up with "The ALS Rules." Many of them focus on the Zen thing of staying in the present moment. I'm not the first to come up with self-help ideas, but I'm happy to share them and have done so at the ALS Clinic and in the next chapter.

Maureen and I are still traveling since I remain able to handle airports and security for now. And at the end of January, we went along with a family member in his private plane for a three-day visit to some friends of his (and now ours) in Hermosillo and Los Mochis, Mexico.

We went down to Phoenix in February to see my son Kevin and his wife Kristen after they recently moved there. That was a six-day trip —the weekend with them and four rounds of golf for us. We have taken several car trips to see Maureen's family in King City and had a short stay in Bodega Bay. We're also thinking about another big vacation this spring and maybe a cruise to Alaska this summer. Most cruise lines are ADA wheelchair accessible, which I'll probably need by that point.

My daily routine is slowing down a bit and contracting since I move and do things much slower than usual. I joke that tasks take me twice as long and three times the energy to accomplish. I usually take off the brace and switch to the walker in the evenings when I'm tired.

I seem to need more sleep than I ever did—ten hours at night and, frequently, a nap in the afternoon. It makes the days seem short and hard to get my to-do list finished, as you can imagine. But having an agenda (one of my rules) and going after it gives my days a focus. Now it's the end of March, and I'm still functioning okay.

TEN

The ALS Rules

~

Author's note: Originally written in December 2006, these rules were periodically modified until December 2007. The final version appears below. The most significant change was to Rule 6, which originally read "Push my limits." Over the holidays, this principle led to weeks of despair exhaustion, and depression for Maureen and me, so I changed it.

I printed these in large type and read them each morning without fail.

1. Don't always follow the rules.
2. Know that ALS doesn't always follow its own rules.
3. Remember that I am not the only one who has my ALS.
4. Focus on what I can do, not what I can't do.
5. Have an agenda for every day.
6. Pace myself (and Maureen).
7. Find ways to laugh as much as possible.
8. Have contact every day with family or friends.
9. Focus on and spend time with positive people and things.
10. Contemplating courage for the rest of my life is overwhelming, but courage for today is possible.

Another copy of "The ALS Rules" is located in Appendix B.

ELEVEN

Transitions: Alaska, Falling, and Using a Wheelchair

~

Well, I'm unsure of this chapter's theme. At first, I was thinking *transitions*, but after my recent UCSF ALS Clinic visit, it seems more like the not-so-good news variety. Maureen came up with a well-phrased synthesis: we are entering the period of *safety and energy conservation.*

But all of these themes, at least in part, seem to convey a negative picture. Although the physical realities are challenging on all levels, I remain mostly (and irrationally) upbeat and happy. Anyway, I'll let you decide. As Joe Friday from the old TV series *Dragnet* insisted, "Just the facts, please."

My breathing is still steady at the 92 percent measurement. My weight is stable, and my nutritionist loves me. My speech was going downhill last spring, so I investigated alternatives and acquired some text-to-speech software for my computer. By now, some of you have heard me use my computer voice. Fortunately, mine has been holding its own for the last few months, so I haven't been forced to use it yet. It's a parlor game trick at this point.

The ALS has now started in my left leg. With the right leg severely affected, my balance is dreadful; the consequence of that progression. I fatigue very quickly with any walking. I fell a few weeks ago, the first time in a year. These days, I can't last for eighteen holes of golf, so it's time to get my first wheelchair. We started using one at airports in July, and though it felt very odd at first, it's well worth it. So this coming week, I'll have a power chair delivered that is a *starter* model. It's somewhat lighter weight, can be disassembled quickly, and is transportable by car. It's designed to help me get around, but not sit in all day.

Dr. Cathy is also giving me some new meds to experiment with, in hopes of reducing both the tension/spasms in my muscles and my cough. I'm still in the high dose CoQ10 study until December, and there may be another study drug after that. But there are still no miracles out there, and I'm not holding my breath for any. Pun intended.

Again, on to the fun stuff! We made several more trips to King City to see Maureen's folks and a couple to Bodega Bay. We even played a little golf with friends a few times on the Bodega Bay course—there are seven holes on the back nine that I can still navigate.

This summer, we traveled to Phoenix for a brief weekend trip to visit my son Kevin and his wife Kristen. We had to check out their first home purchase in a suburb called Gilbert. Fortunately, we hit cooler weather—it was only 110 degrees! My daughter Carey came up for five days earlier this month. It was another great visit.

Our big trip was a ten-day cruise to Alaska in late July. We sailed in and out of San Francisco. It was a marvelous experience; we saw glaciers, nature's beauty, and lots of wildlife. The funniest thing was encountering Bob and Goldie Delsman when we boarded—former patients who sailed with us. Maureen and I enjoyed getting to know them as friends now. We've been showing people my DVD production of the photos Maureen took.

We're getting good use out of our house on Vista Del Mundo which is ideal for entertaining visitors. A lot of family and friends have visited, staying over in the "west wing" and enjoying the positive energy our house and deck have to offer. One highlight was the weekend we had a houseful of family over, and I was asked to throw the first pitch at the Sacramento River Cats baseball game.

As I said at the beginning of this chapter, this is a transition time for me/us. I have had three years where my life was not just about ALS—it was about doing most of the things I have wanted to do while maneuvering around the progressing problems. I am entering a period where the disabilities are catching up with me, impacting my ability to walk, drive, and play golf. As a substitute, I'm expanding my computer and DVD production skills and enjoying the creative outlet.

Now more than ever, "The ALS Rules" are coming into play. The priority is focusing on what I can do (rather than what I can't). At the top of my daily list is having frequent contact with family and friends and keeping the laughter coming. Speaking of which—did you hear about the Irishman who walked out of a bar?

It really happened.

TWELVE

I Take Away My Own Keys

~

I went to UCSF for a visit in December 2007. I've been very lucky to have ALS (Excuse me, would you mind repeating that?) for three years. I still worked for two of them, played golf, kept driving, and pretty much carried on as usual until last September.

Well, I'm no longer driving. Let me tell you about that. Going to REI in the spring of 2006 and buying a hiking stick to use as a cane was another emotional blow to the gut. It was my first visible admission that something was wrong with me. It was relatively easy with the driving. I didn't want to have to explain to a cop why I was still driving with ALS in my leg and arm after having just t-boned a school bus.

I'm unable to walk much, so I mostly live in a power wheelchair. I'm also having a lot of trouble speaking, so I just got a great speech-generating touchscreen device. I expect to be relying on it more and more as I learn how to use it.

I sound like the time I had three beers during an afternoon of golf, a margarita after the round, two scotches before dinner, and most of a bottle of wine one night (my share) at a brothers' weekend. If I talked loudly enough and used words that can't be printed, my brothers understood me just fine. First, because we're Irish, and second, they all were way ahead of me.

My breathing number is down from 92 percent to 84. Both the respiratory therapist and I think it's because my darn palate is flopping around like a fish with the hook still in its lip. They want me to have another nocturnal oxygen test to make sure I'm still breathing okay when asleep (not imitating one of those dead frogs in high school biology).

My left arm and hand are still unaffected so far, and my grip strength in the right hand is still strong more than three years later. From a safety standpoint, this is wonderful news. No falls since August (knock on wood).

Many people saw me out in public with the new lightweight wheelchair, but it turned out I'm too big for this type. I look like Fred Flintstone in a Mini Cooper. So, I'm in a larger model now (a Permobil C300, if you want to google it). I have a loaner until my custom-fit chair arrives, hopefully by February. We'll need to buy a special van to go anywhere because it won't collapse and fit in our car like the other one.

I haven't played golf in six weeks or so, but there's a slim chance that a second left leg brace may give me enough balance and strength to hack away a few more times when it arrives. I now dig a divot so big—they follow me around with bright orange hazard cones to warn the golfers behind me.

It's December 2007, and we're in the midst of an enjoyable holiday season. My kids and family are visiting. After that, we'll be starting the serious business of turning our plan for the master bathroom remodel into reality. The trick is making it accessible for what I'll need, but still be attractive. Hopefully, it won't take too long because, while I'm safe in the shower for the time being, I'm a definite risk, as in the "Help! I've fallen, and I can't get up!" commercial.

THIRTEEN

Ozzie and Harriet Beds

~

We finally finished our bathroom remodel this past April, so we're back in the master suite. I can use the bathroom I designed, and there are no more nicks (to understate it) in the guest room doorways. It's beautiful, yet functional; it will accommodate my needs to the end. I'll be modest and say I should receive some kind of award from the American Architectural Association or a Nobel Prize. At least I deserve a write-up in the AARP magazine. I'm expecting a call any day now.

I can get in and safely use the toilet, shower, and sink. I'm still independent in there, although I can sense the clock is ticking. The other revolutionary change is that we're both sleeping better since I broke down and agreed to have a (separate) hospital bed with a trapeze. I miss reaching over in bed and copping a socially acceptable feel—especially in the mornings, if you catch my drift. I am sad to report: we are both happier, we sleep better, and we realize how my thrashing around was making us both sleep-deprived.

We went to the ALS Clinic in May, but the news was mostly bad, so piss on it. My breathing number took another drop to 73 percent. You may remember I started four years ago at 98 percent, and it held in the nineties until a year ago, when I started falling off the cliff. My diaphragm remains strong, so I'm not yet ready for a BiPAP machine to help me breathe at night when I'm heavily sedated. BiPAP uses a mask, not a tracheostomy tube (which I've declined). Apparently, the BiPAP recommendation comes when you have more symptoms or hit the 50 percent number. I actually won't be surprised if that's within the year.

My right arm and both legs continue to weaken slowly, and the ALS has finally appeared in my left arm. My speech is now going downhill fast. On a positive note, I can curse someone up one side and down the other, and they just say, "Huh?" The doctor was mainly concerned about my progressively worsening stiffness despite high doses of Valium and another muscle relaxer. I'll be a zombie when I check out. "Paging Betty Ford." That's okay with me.

At the end of the day, Dr. Cathy spontaneously launched into a discussion about hospice and ways to keep me comfortable at the end, when I will no longer eat or take meds by mouth. It later struck Maureen and me as odd this conversation didn't make us feel scared, frightened, or surprised. I'm not afraid of dying—it's the dependence on others for personal care that's distressing to contemplate. But that's my fate.

The latest thing I have had to accept is the loss of golf. I tried a few outings in February and March, but by April, I really couldn't hit the ball at all and fell once, so that was that. The clubs are in storage, and we sold our membership in the golf club.

On a brighter note, we took an eight-day road trip to Phoenix to visit my son Kevin and his wife Kristen. We had a good time and saw a lot of sights. We had fairly good luck with the ADA accommodations in the hotels. Even so, we discovered that with my *issues,* it's now too hard for both of us. Too many hours in the car meant leg problems for me, and neither of us got good sleep. So, no more long road trips. And air travel is out—I can't trust the airlines with my chair (too risky). At this point, we're planning on mostly staying and sleeping at home except for one or two night trips for special occasions and not too far away.

If this seems like a huge change from my March appointment, it is. In the early days of 2005 and 2006, I was working, traveling, and golfing. The ALS was there but didn't limit me/us too much. Not much changed from month to month. Now all my reserve capacity is gone, and every little bit of muscle loss hits me harder. It seems I'm changing faster. That's what makes me sometimes mutter incomprehensible expletives to people who see me and routinely comment, "You look so good."

I feel like saying, "Are you blind? I am in a wheelchair, mostly paralyzed, and can't talk!"

I guess I understand their problem. What are they supposed to say? I look like I could stand up and walk any minute. But the truth is—I can't.

So, I make a joke.

FOURTEEN

How to Frighten Your Caregiver

~

We hired a paid caregiver to help me in the mornings when Maureen isn't here. The duties are pretty light right now—set up the bathroom, lay out my clothes, make me breakfast, and mainly be here in case of—"Help! I've fallen, and I can't get up!"

Maureen went to Stanford with her dad this morning, and Bonita (Spanish for, "Everyone should have one of her") was here. And no, she isn't twenty-three and doesn't look like Catherine Zeta-Jones. Do you think Maureen is crazy?

My first order of business is to take care of duties in "the reading room." That's where guys go in the morning, turn on the fan, and um—read. Currently, I have a book in there that's a collection of Dave Barry columns. Dave is an award-winning syndicated writer for the *Miami Herald,* and he is a funny, funny guy. This anthology is entitled *Boogers Are My Beat.* I'm reading one of his columns about the 2002 Winter Olympics in Salt Lake City, and I start laughing.

Unfortunately, when ALS affects your tongue and everything within four inches thereof, your laughter mostly sounds like a mule gagging on a kielbasa sausage—the echo in a small room is spectacular.

I am in there, all bodily functions are loudly out of control, and poor Bonita understandably gets worried. She knocks and asks, "Are you all right in there?" When is the last time someone knocked on *your* door and asked that when *you* were in the crapper?

I managed to gasp that I was okay and would explain later—when my pants weren't around my ankles. Lucky for me, she's taken care of a number of demented patients over the years and will come back.

Oh, I forgot to mention that the first thing I did when I started laughing was empty my nasal contents. So, anyone who wants to look at the book next time they visit will want to wear gloves.

FIFTEEN

I Turn Fifty-Four

~

I just turned fifty-four the day before my UCSF appointment on March 21, 2008. Maureen broke protocol and threw me a surprise party. She had thrown a big surprise bash for me on my fiftieth, so I thought I was done with surprises. But this was nice—very low-key, just a dozen close friends dropping by after work. It was great to see them all.

At UCSF, I told the staff that I was functionally a lot better than in December because of my custom-fit wheelchair. It finally arrived in January and has made a world of difference—where I can go and what I can do. I had a loaner in December, but it caused my legs to go numb. If you can't move them, it's quite irritating.

We just purchased a wheelchair-modified minivan and are ready for a road trip or two this spring while I can still handle ADA hotel rooms and bathrooms. The good news is that I'm sleeping better since we kicked the cats out of the bedroom, got an air purifier, and I started some meds to keep my nose clear at night. I can breathe again! Medical note: breathing is important.

I let the staff know that there was minimal change in my legs and right hand/arm. With help, I'm still able to stand up from the chair or pull on something nearby. I take care of myself in the bathroom and shower. I can dress myself and put on the clunky shoes/braces, but it's hard and takes forever, so I appreciate the occasional help.

I've developed some edema (water swelling) in both legs and an ulcer on my toe, so from the knees down—except for the lack of a kilt—I look like the character, Fat Bastard, from the Austin Powers movies. To paraphrase Fat Bastard, "I am one sexy beast" from the legs on down.

I did get a second AFO brace, this one for my left leg. With that to help my balance and stamina, I've gone back out with my buddies to the golf course—the first time since November. My swing would make Ben Hogan roll over in his grave, and I'm very limited in what I can do, but I guess anything is better than nothing. The groundskeepers and fellow golfers are drinking more than usual. They thought they were rid of me.

The other big news around here is that we've been living in the guest bedroom for more than six weeks now since the bathroom is being remodeled to accommodate the wheelchair. My chair and I have put some gouges in the narrow doorways. It looks like I used a pickaxe. We had to move out of the entire master suite because the area looks like a cruise missile strike zone.

I decided to put myself on an experimental drug for ALS in February. Lithium has been around for thirty years or so to treat bipolar mania. Recently, some Italian researchers did a small study showing great promise with ALS and a low lithium dose. It supposedly slowed or stopped progression. There were a lot of trials in the planning stages, but they would take months to get going, and I was running out of time. This lithium follow-up experiment was worldwide, internet-based, and overseen by someone with a scientific background. So I thought, "Why not?" Unfortunately, like all the rest, lithium didn't work.

Occasionally, something really gratifying happens that cheers me up, like my sister's cover article on me in the *Sacramento News and Review* issue (February 7, 2008), or a music concert, or playing golf, or the surprise party. But those can't happen every day for any of us. So, each day is its own story.

SIXTEEN

Tina

~

I guess when dinner is a scotch and appetizers, the rest of the evening shouldn't be a surprise. But even I might not believe what I'm about to tell you if Maureen hadn't been there to bear witness. In fact, she encouraged some of the players. Yes, there were several, but one will linger in my memory for some time; she was the first and the best, and her name was Tina.

I was acting like a cranky SOB one morning, so Maureen booked me an early birthday surprise—tickets to see Wayman Tisdale and Michael Lington at the Radisson the next night. She also booked a room, so we could stay after the show.

For those who don't know of him, Wayman, at that time, was on his second very successful career, leading a smooth jazz band as a bass player after retiring as a six-nine power forward in the NBA (playing for the Sacramento Kings, no less!). That cheered me up pretty well. Unfortunately, he has since died of cancer—a huge loss of a great and talented man.

We arrived there early, checked in, and thought we'd grab a quick bite in the bar so that we'd arrive early for the show. Scotch on the rocks, wine for Maureen, a quesadilla, and some chicken tenders sounded *really* tasty—you know what I mean?

We got to the ballroom early. The wheelchair area was supposed to be the first row of general admission seats behind the reserved section, way back, but what's the other option? It turned out the entire first row was full, well over an hour before show time. We were cruising around, looking for space, looking for an usher. Then along came Tina.

First, Tina is cute. Quite an eyeful. She's maybe forty-something, a tall, attractive, black woman with blonde dreadlocks, dressed in tight red leather pants and a red top. Oh, and she is totally blitzed. I mean *totally.* She's full of personality and having a great time just wandering around, looking for action—when she spies us. Tina takes a liking to me, Maureen laughingly strikes up a conversation, and Tina decides to take me on as her project—finding me a better seat.

Tina's method of doing this is looking around as she repeatedly puts her hands on me (squeezing my shoulders, rubbing my head, giving me hugs—you get the idea). Her dreadlocks are constantly in my face when she talks to me. She bestows several kisses on me, and when Maureen compliments her on the red leather pants, Tina throws one leg in my lap and offers to give them to her because they'd fit her. At that moment, Tina is the most entertaining, delightful woman I have ever met in my life—except my wife, of course.

So there I am, having a marvelous time, and the show hasn't even started. When has *this* ever happened? We're all laughing because my wife is egging her on, and I'm enjoying the show. Maureen goes off to find an usher, leaving me alone with Tina. What she said to me is not ready for publication.

Maureen returns with Fritz, a nice balding guy already looking harried an hour before the show. Tina wastes no time getting up in his grill about finding me a better seat. I can see the wheels grinding away as he tries to make sense of this picture of the three of us—a middle-aged white couple, the man's in a wheelchair with a sexy black chick doing a lap dance on him. Maureen finally explains that it's just the two of us; Tina already has a seat with her girlfriends. She goes off with Fritz to find a spot when the girlfriends show up—two pleasant black ladies about my age, more conservatively and nicely dressed. They say, "Hello," then walk quickly away to their seats. Tina doesn't leave my side until Maureen returns. Fritz has gotten us great seats closer to the stage against the wall. We regrettably bid her adieu, and she sashays off on another adventure.

We take our places against the wall, and Maureen leaves to find me another scotch. Why not? Pretty soon here comes Fritz with Enoch, another guy in a wheelchair. Enoch is an unfortunate fellow who was in an auto accident in 1995. He had a traumatic left-brain injury that left him with impaired movement on the right side and difficulty speaking (my diagnosis).

Fritz puts them on the wall just in front of us, but that's fine because the stage is way off to our side. Enoch looks about thirty and is accompanied by his sister Tracey, who spends a lot of time talking with Maureen as they are sitting adjacent to each other.

Then, the show starts, and I can highly recommend Michael Lington—a Danish-born sax player with a killer band who knows how to entertain. He plays for a bit over an hour and gets everybody going. When Wayman comes out, the crowd is ready to party. He says, "It's nice to be home," since his music career started while he was playing for the Sacramento Kings. Everyone roars. Anyway, here begins part two of my story which involves a wide side aisle, great music, and people who want to dance. One gal named Christine especially stands out. She's a good-looking thirty-something brunette in a nice jacket with sparkles from Nordstrom (Maureen asked), pants, and high heels. Unlike Tina, Christine isn't loaded, but she's having a great time. Can you guess where this is going?

Everyone is standing, so I have the chair up to full height (eight inches extra) to see. I'm trying to get a groove going in my wheelchair—I'm feeling it (the second scotch?)—and Christine decides to dance with me.

So she grabs my hands, dances with me, and as she gets close, I see Maureen is struggling with whether to laugh or keel over from shock. I'm glad I had turned the power off on the chair because part of her dance is to caress my joystick (on the wheelchair control, I mean). When the song ends, Christine gives me a hug and a kiss, tells me how great I am, then goes back to her seat by her husband. Maureen is staring at me, laughing, but we're not done yet.

Enoch is feeling the groove also, but all he can do is sway his head and raise his left arm, God bless him. But there's this big guy in a bright orange shirt and pants sitting on the end of a row across from us. He's been up dancing by himself (I suspect his wife won't join him because he's also really lit up). So he comes over to me, offers to buy me a drink, then walks down the line asking Maureen, then Tracey, then Enoch, who mumbles, "Corona!"

Mr. Orange Shirt ends up buying Enoch two Coronas which makes his sister Tracey say nervously to Maureen, "I'm in trouble—our mother doesn't let Enoch drink at all!" He also buys Enoch a CD. He is truly a generous human being.

When the music starts again, we're all doing our version of dancing. Mr. Orange Shirt comes over, grabs my hands, and dances with me. He doesn't go near the joystick, so I'm okay with it. Getting down with Wayman, it's just joyous moving to good music. He dances with Enoch and Tracey, and Maureen a bit also. But as the song is ending, he is back at my end of the line. And I kid you not, he leans over and kisses me on the cheek, then goes to sit by his wife.

When Maureen gets her eyeballs back in their sockets, she says, "What *is* it with you tonight?"

I say, "I don't know. Maybe it's the big, black, sexy wheelchair; maybe it's because I'm alert, not drooling, can move a bit, and am *totally* non-threatening."

But here are two things I know: we need to get out more, and I'm drinking more scotch when we do. I'm glad we had a hotel room right there down the hallway for the night. It came in handy.

SEVENTEEN

Music and Dancing

On Saturday, Maureen and I went down the hill to a graduation party, then met some friends for dinner, so it turned into a pleasant yet long day. Lately, all this means is no nap for me. I went to bed exhausted and slept in a bit Sunday morning. I was on the verge of second-guessing our plans to go down the hill for the Sacramento Jazz Festival.

We haven't been for a few years, so we made plans. We've always enjoyed it—mostly seeing blues, zydeco, and swing band acts. Anyone who enjoys live music and lives in the area (or even if you don't) should plan to go see it sometime.

Anyway, we arrived at the Sacramento Convention Center venue area about 11:30 a.m. We picked that site because it was more likely to be accessible to me in the wheelchair. There were at least six separate stages at the center including the Hyatt and the Sheraton. The first positive omen was that we got a two-for-one deal on the tickets. Then, after looking at the program, we raced over to the Hyatt ballroom to catch one of the featured bands, Tom Rigney and Flambeau.

The show was underway in front of a packed auditorium of more than a thousand, but an usher took us up front, and we ended up in a wheelchair space with an empty companion seat. They play mostly zydeco, some blues, and one song sounded almost Irish (we found out he has some green ancestors). It was a great show.

Then, we went back to the convention center for a quick lunch and proceeded to dash around and see most of the six acts and brief snippets of two others in seven hours. That's how we roll. But that wasn't why we stayed there until 8:00 p.m.—way past when we had planned. It was—the dancing. They had dance floors by the side of every stage at the Jubilee. In the main hall at the convention center, there was a huge floor in front of the bandstand with bleachers set up on each side. The reason for this: there was a swing dance competition. I never knew that.

I don't watch that TV show with the dancing. Even though the costumes the gals wear would get you arrested for being a streetwalking hooker in most major metropolitan areas, I have zero interest. That shouldn't come as a shock to those who know me well. ALS does nothing to interfere with your sex drive—which eventually presents certain difficulties, as you can imagine.

When we were passing through the hall at 2:00 p.m., we got a glimpse of the activity going on, and we were fascinated and hooked. That venue was set up for the big band/swing band acts, and there were innumerable good dancers on and off the floor all afternoon and evening. We would come and go, and I could always score a wheelchair spot right up front. We listened to some great big bands and watched incredibly talented dancers do their thing.

Apparently, there are a couple of local clubs, and I guess they all come out for this day every year. Young and old, elegant in spats, dresses, or jeans and sneakers, they could move! We tried to guess their stories: "Is that one a professional? That couple must be in their late seventies. That Asian kid dancing with his mother can't be ten years old! How can he be so good?" The athleticism combined with the rhythm of the twenty-somethings was riveting.

We'd walk over to the Hyatt and see Zydeco Flames and drink a margarita, then meander back to the music of the 1940s, energetically danced to by kids in their twenties, then go upstairs for a glimpse of Igor and his Jazz Cowboys (he's a real pro and funny).

We were finally feeling tired and ready to head home at six-thirty when we realized the dance finals competition was at seven. They were dancing to a band called Evolution from North Bend, Oregon (composed of high schoolers and at least one kid who was still in eighth grade!). How was this going to work? Maureen looked at me, I looked at her, and we decided to stay. As they called the eight finalist couples for the dance-off, we realized we'd hardly seen any of them on the floor in the previous few hours! We'd been watching and were wowed by the local amateurs! A thousand dollar prize and some airline tickets (Southwest was the sponsor) were on the line. These people were serious and used to performing for a crowd, so I got the impression there might be a circuit, but I could be wrong.

I needn't have wondered about the band. The musicians are pros with a website (http://www.labband.com/new/index.php), four CDs, and a touring schedule. They ripped through some standards like nobody's business and at a breakneck tempo. We saw some even more spectacular dancing and were awed by the kids in the band. It was 8:00 p.m., and we were hungry and an hour from home.

Fortunately for us, Mikuni Restaurant (sushi) was on the next block, so we had a light dinner and arrived home a little after ten. Having been gone twelve hours, we were both exhausted, and I was off my medicine schedule. My swollen feet were killing me, but we were very, very glad we went. So, I'll rest today and tomorrow while Maureen is busy. It's time for lunch and a nap.

EIGHTEEN

Friday the 13th

This series of events happened to me on Friday the 13th, but time means little to me now. It was my own fault, of course. Early in the morning after my shower, I was sitting there naked in the bathroom, watching my caregiver dry off my shriveled wienie. She mentioned what day it was and asked if I was superstitious to which I replied, "No." What an idiot!

First, let me give you a little background. Well, miracle of miracles, I finally *did* prove to Medicare that I qualify for our tax dollars to get me that BiPAP machine (not a ventilator). This machine helps people like me with ALS continue to breathe deeply through the night when I have enough muscle relaxers on board to put down an African bull elephant. It blows air up your nose (and no, there is no cocaine attachment option).

At first, they gave me the mask option (not the nasal pillows—those came later and worked much better). Fitting the BiPAP mask properly is tricky and looks scary to a layperson. Maureen was gone when the delivery arrived, so my brothers Greg and David, who were staying the night, got the unexpected shock of seeing me in my Darth Vader disguise ("Come to the Dark Side!"). If they wet their pants, they kept it from me; God bless them.

So anyway, the thing delivers humidified air, and it comes with a heater. For a few nights, it seemed too hot to me, so I had Maureen leave the heater off—on Friday the 13th, of course (some people used to think I was smart). All was well until bedtime, when some idiot (me again) unwittingly backed the wheelchair onto the electric blanket control.

I didn't sleep well that night, to put it mildly. First off, I had a nightmare that the house was on fire and awoke to find the blanket temperature feeling about 900 degrees. So, I quietly (to not awaken Maureen) took fifteen minutes to manipulate the bed and with one hand pull the blanket off most of my upper body. Then, I fell asleep.

I dreamt that I was part of Captain Scott's Antarctic expedition and awoke to frigidly cold air blowing up my nose. So, I tried (quietly again) to turn off the machine and take off the mask. But this time, Maureen got up, looked at the mess I'd made, and said, "What the heck are you doing?" It was probably three o'clock in the morning, so I told Maureen what had happened. She discovered that my wheelchair's tire had turned the electric blanket dial from low to "bake at 350 degrees for eight hours." She fixed that, and I had her turn the humidifier heat back to low. She reconnected the BiPAP, and I finally went back to sleep.

By then, the night was ruined, and I felt terrorized by what would happen next. Well, I awoke with an infected toe (paronychia, if you want to look it up). Fortunately, the toe infection was in the early stage, and the physician had healed himself by the next day.

But I'm not finished. I had managed to (privately, thank God) embarrass myself earlier on Friday when Maureen showed me a gift her mom had given her on a recent visit. It was about ten inches long, cylindrical, and battery powered. (Wait a minute! I know I'm in a wheelchair, but Maureen doesn't talk about sex to *anybody*, especially her mother!) Then she says, "It's a wine bottle cork remover." I felt like an idiot. Unfortunately, this is a familiar feeling, even as I age.

So, the next time Friday the 13th rolls around, I think I'll just stay in bed and pull the covers over my head.

NINETEEN

ALS Improves Your Golf

~

The fault, dear Brutus, is not in our star but in ourselves …

—William Shakespeare

Well, at least this applies to golf.

We need to do a little time warp here because as I write this, I haven't played in nearly two years. But I had to put this chapter in somewhere, and so far, I think this book is boring. So, I will lead you through the agony and ecstasy (using the sports cliché) of the adventures during the first few years with Lou Gehrig's disease.

I'm a slow learner when it comes to sports. I played organized, referee basketball from age ten to forty-two, but I never learned the proper technique (or had the arm strength) for shooting a free throw until I was in my thirties.

I started waterskiing late in my twenties, and it took years for me to learn to get up on one ski (slalom ski). Soon after, I was cutting back and forth on a competition course with buoys while using a fifteen-foot shortened rope and having great fun. I wasn't very skilled, but I did it.

I took up snow skiing at age thirty or so (a big mistake) when we moved near the mountains. I spent years going ass-over-teakettle on the green slopes (the easiest) until I finally got it one vacation while using the new parabolic skis. In four days, I went from green slopes to black diamond. I kid you not. So, you get the idea. Apparently, I didn't, because I seriously started playing and trying to learn golf in my forties. What a bonehead.

Golf is a game invented by sadistic Scots who named it that since the other four-letter word that starts with "F" was already taken.

They perversely ended the name of their game with that letter, obviously just for spite. Scots.

I had played in the local hospital's charity tournament, which was a scramble format. I would miraculously hit one good shot for my foursome all day, drink beer, and enjoy the party afterward. Then, one day, after playing a course with three strangers, I was so bad that I drove straight to the hospice charity store and gave them all my clubs and equipment.

A year went by, and the goddamn tournament was looming again. So, I foolishly signed up for a series of lessons, bought some proper clubs for my height (nearly six feet four), and got serious. I read books. I read magazine articles. I learned what you *should* do—and it started working. I didn't cheat on my scorecard (much), and over the next few years, my handicap index went from the high thirties to twenty-seven, to twenty-four, to nineteen. I even had a legitimate, well-hit, not totally lucky hole-in-one. I convinced myself that I could eventually reach a respectable ten handicap or so.

Then I decided to get ALS. I'd probably have only three to five years to live, not even considering how long I'd be on my feet and out of a wheelchair. So, I had a brilliant idea—let's spend (waste) thousands of dollars and join a country club. Now I can play golf all the time! And we did.

I started working in earnest on the finer points of my game: the slice, the shank. I rolled a twenty-foot downhill putt ten feet past the hole with the ball waving merrily as it raced by.

My right hand, the first to go, cost me immediately (when you hit a golf ball for distance, you need that snap in your wrists at the very end of the swing—like when you shoot a free throw or use a whip). Starting in 2004, I had no snap, so I had shorter and shorter distances with every club.

But despite that, from June 2004 until April 2008, when I played for the last time, I enjoyed every round, every second, every dirty joke, and every *nineteenth hole* more than ever before. I tried to describe it to my buddies, but it was hard for them to fully understand.

There are two stories from that time I need to share. One is a life lesson, one makes me laugh to this day. Every private golf club has an annual invitational member-guest tournament, wherein the member invites a non-member friend to join him in a multi-day competition with lots of booze, prizes, booze, parties, booze, food, side bets, and booze—did I mention that? Of course, it's a thinly-veiled recruitment tool, but a lot of fun and only sets you back several hundred dollars to participate. Just after I retired on April 30, 2006, I signed up for my one and only tournament with Mark Kal (my friend, doctor, and oh, yes, an excellent golfer). There were about seventy teams.

One of the side competitions was the two-man putting contest, held on the first day with tee off at seven sharp. Now keep in mind, I had just retired from a scaled-back job because I could barely make it through a ten-hour (shortened) day. So, I got up at four-thirty to get ready, meet up with Mark, drive to the course, and warm up.

They held the qualifier for the putting contest (to qualify for the elimination bracket) in the afternoon, and we squeaked in. Then, we heard the good news: the completion wouldn't start until after dinner that night. Not nearly enough time to go home and grab a quick nap, so we dropped by our nearby office, gloated about golfing while they were working, then went back to the club and chilled for a few hours.

Fred, the assistant pro at the club, ran this sideshow, and he had heard through the grapevine (a secret at the club) that I had ALS. His uncle had died of it, so he knew the score. Fred set up a nine-hole course on the practice green with ten to fifteen-foot putts uphill, downhill, breaking sidehill, etc.

The teams had been slashed to sixteen by the qualifier. The format was alternate shot, with the member putting first on the odd holes (one, three, five, etc.). It was getting dark after dinner, so they had set up floodlights for us.

After we won our first match, I told Freddie, and he (knowing I'd been there all day) said, "Great!" Under his breath, he asked how I was holding up. I said that I was okay, and we awaited our next opponent. He was quite surprised when we won again and got to the semifinals.

Freddie saw that I was weak and not so subtly using my putter as a cane to walk around. He asked if he could get me a chair, but I declined because, of course, that would have indicated weakness.

It was past eight and getting dark when we discovered our next opponents were fifty to sixtyish serious golfers, and the member was a patient of Mark's. They were good putters. I mean *really* good putters. For some reason, I'd been doing pretty well all day (e.g., I drained the last ten-foot putt that got us through the qualifier). I hit a terrible first putt on hole one; we lost the hole, and I said to myself, "Well, just like me—saving my worst for last."

Standing at hole two and watching Mark hit first, I realized what I had done mentally to myself. What a guaranteed way to lose! I decided, goddammit, I wanted to *win* this thing. So I did a mental about-face and got better. By now, a crowd was watching. Still, we went two down before I holed out three successive shots, breaking twelve to fifteen-foot putts on five, seven, and nine to beat them, one-up. Mark was in shock, and Freddie couldn't believe it.

The finals were anti-climactic. It was twice around (eighteen holes), and the other guys were in their thirties. We trounced them, five up with four holes left to play! It was almost 9:00 p.m. I'd had ALS in my right arm for two years now and in my right leg for a year, and I'd been up (mostly on my feet) for sixteen hours.

My trophy sits in the living room—a very pretty gold-engraved magnum of cabernet sauvignon (which we drank at the family reunion in August that summer). Of course, the lesson is the incredible power of the mind and will over the body. Two nights later, my hardest remaining challenge was walking up a grassy hill with the full bottle in the dark after the awards ceremony. I refused to fall. By then, I had been using a cane for two months, although not at the golf club.

But the best memory I have of the three days was hole fifteen (the third day, I think). It was an alternate-shot format that day, and fifteen is a straightforward par-five birdie opportunity. Of course, the PGA guys hit a three-wood and wedge to the green for an eagle, but they were obviously from another planet. So I hit a decent drive (for me) into the fairway—but by that time, I only made it about 200 yards downrange. Mark hit a spectacular three-wood to the middle of the fairway, eighty yards from the green. That's when the fun started.

Previously that day, Mark put a drive (after an unlucky bounce) into a grass drainage ditch, so I shanked it about fifty yards into a fairway sand trap. He'd had a hole-in-one on a par four. The hole he hit was into a ladies' purse under the fairway tree he nicked (of course, golf *does* have a rule for that). The entire day was going that way, and our playing partners were starting to think we were mortal enemies, not best friends.

So back to hole fifteen. I had eighty yards into a flat green, an easy wedge shot. Naturally, I pulled it left into a deep greenside sand trap. As I said before, Mark is an excellent golfer, but somewhere in his primordial reptilian brain he was thinking, "Payback time." His bunker shot sailed over the green toward a creek on the other side.

I looked and realized it was not in the *hazard* (creek), but on the dirt under a tree with some branches piled up in front of it. The rules allow you to move debris piled for removal, so I did and got ready to punch the ball onto the green.

I noticed the ground was moving under my feet. I was standing on an ant hill, and they were upset about it for some reason. I quickly hit the ball, and we two-putted for a double bogey while our playing partners rolled on the ground, laughing. I swatted at ants on my shoes, socks, and legs for the next two holes. I swear, I'm not making any of this up. Well, maybe the part about them rolling around on the ground. But all the rest is true.

After two years with the ALS, my handicap (I still recorded scores at that time) soared back to the stratosphere, and even with Mark's skill, my one goal was not to finish last. We didn't. We finished sixty-sixth out of seventy. It cost the other four teams a whole lot of money to keep me from putting their names here.

The last time I went out was April 2008. By then, I was in my first portable wheelchair and wore braces on both legs. My buddies had to hold me up while I transferred from the car to the golf cart. Back on the course, they helped me walk to the ball, teed up for me, then stood back when I got my balance. We called it *valet golf.* I could hit my driver maybe a hundred yards. I'd hit a few shots, land close or on the green, then have them pick up the ball for me.

On the last day, Jon Lehrman set me up for a fairway shot and stood back. I topped the ball, it rolled maybe fifty yards, and as I looked up to watch, I lost my balance. I slowly fell forward on my face like a giant redwood. I could just imagine a logger yelling, "Tim-ber!"

They managed to get me back on my feet and into the cart, but I was a little shaken and done with that hole. Minutes later, I teed off on the next hole and finished the round with Jon and Steve Green (who felt unnecessarily guilty for not catching me). Since I hadn't hit the ball well all day, I decided that was it. Maureen stopped playing as well, so we sold our membership.

TWENTY

Constipation

~

Now there's a catchy title! Maybe it makes you want to take this piece of paper, unread, and use it to line the birdcage. Or maybe not. Maybe you're in that demographic (like us) who watches the evening news and are alternately bombarded by commercials for products that turn your female bladder into cast iron, make your prostate flow like the Hoover Dam outlet, or make a fifty-five-year-old guy's hair so irresistible, that Victoria's Secret models want to get in his pants. Or maybe you think, pray, and hope that I, as a certified medical doctor, have solved a problem that will win me the Nobel Prize for medicine.

As you know, ALS is medical shorthand for "You drew the short straw." But you've got to look for the positives, so I thought I might help my impacted brethren with these simple words of advice: Dave Barry.

His columns are so successful that he now makes money selling books of his columns (dating back to 1827, or something). Buy them. He is a funny, funny guy. But enough about him, let's talk about me.

The human body is a marvel. All pieces and parts are meant to act in concert until we put a bullet in it somewhere or make a routine out of supersizing our McDonald's order. But part of the equation is that you're able to walk around.

As you more astute observers have noticed, I've grown lazy and mostly ride around in a wheelchair which the American taxpayers of 2023 bought for me last year. This transition had numerous unintended consequences, a concept which anyone who may follow government legislation is very familiar. For instance, bladder spasms come with ALS. They remind me of the cold war drills of the 1960s, wherein once a month, a siren went off in your city and all of you fourth graders had five seconds to crawl under your desk and kiss your ass goodbye.

Anyway, these spasms are a bit inconvenient when I'm sitting in the living room recliner and get the two-minute warning from the bladder area. It takes me what seems like forever to transfer to the wheelchair, make it to the bathroom, and eventually reach the stand-up/zipper-down position in close proximity to the porcelain receptacle.

Thankfully, they have a drug that reduces these spasms, but it also decreases the forcefulness of my stream to the point where I need a Viagra to get the water past my toenails. But I digress—we're supposed to be talking about bowels here. Maybe I'll write another piece later on about what happens to certain parts when a guy sits on them all day and they don't get proper exercise, shall we say, for a year or two.

So back to our topic. When you don't walk, you tend to get bound up, as my grandma used to say. And if you're a typical man, there is a certain regularity that develops in the morning, after you've had some coffee and before you shower, that starts the day off on the right foot. You just don't feel right without it. You can't overeat at lunch, find yourself prone to road rage, and are cranky with the staff.

Therefore, as a learned member of the medical profession, it didn't shock me when I eventually developed this malady. After months of trying to change my diet, and do it the natural way, I succumbed to medical solutions.

There are all kinds of pills for this, and I ought to know, having prescribed them 145,769 times in my career. Of course, I promptly took an overdose (because I'm a bloody doctor and know better) and got diarrhea. Go back three paragraphs and change the waste material scenario. Picture yourself in the bathroom, using your cell phone occasionally to call your wife in the den and say, "Clean-up on aisle 7."

And God forbid, there is a comedy on TV as you're standing when transferring to your wheelchair. Unfortunately, laughing seems to inactivate whatever sphincter you most need at the moment. It's one of God's little jokes. These are the things that make life special no matter the circumstances. It had reached the point when my helpful eighty-two-year-old mother-in-law sent me her spare bottles of Imodium, thank you very much.

This went back and forth for a couple of months, and I tried stopping various meds to no avail. My bowels didn't know if it was Tuesday or Cleveland. In the pharmacy, I started to cruise the "Oops! I crapped my pants!" aisle. But I don't want to go there yet, you know? Eventually, I may have to put up with *those* as well, but all in good time. Jeez, I was still playing golf not that long ago.

I may have found an answer. Even knowing that all solutions are temporary with ALS, it's nice to have them for a while. So, I have abandoned all stool softeners, fiber, small doses of Redi-Mix concrete, and all manner of sensible remedies. I now eat whatever I want. And every morning, whether I feel the need or not—I take a seat on the throne and pick up my trusty toilet-side Dave Barry volume. I read a column from one of his books, start laughing hysterically, and voila!

Whatever is in my rectum (anything south of the Mason-Dixon Line), clears out of Dodge like an Olympic sprinter, sometimes with the explosive force of an Atlas rocket. Depending on the column I'm reading, be it gas, liquid, solid, or within a city block of the exit sign, out it comes. Then, I'm good for the day.

Thank you, Dave Barry, wherever you are. I know you've played guitar in several rock bands over the years, so I have a new name for your next one—Empty Rectums. I doubt it's already taken.

TWENTY-ONE

No More Lipstick for the Pig

~

It's November 2008, and I'm facing a challenge. I'm all out of lipstick for the curly-tailed creature in the house that goes, "Oink!" Now, as a friend put it, I have to try and spray-paint a turd. Most days, I just can't, but I'll give it a try.

I'll start with the details everyone always wants. We were just at the ALS Clinic in September. I've only lost a few pounds despite my progressive swallowing difficulties. That made them happy at UCSF, but since I can't exercise, I look like Jabba the Hutt.

My breathing is doing okay, which turns out to be a mixed blessing, but my FRS (functional rating score) continues to drop. It measures things like, "Do you get yourself dressed?" I wonder how they deal with nudists. Things like this keep me up at night.

Steven, Maureen's brother, put it well when he told her that for a long time, "We made it look too easy." But those who have stayed with us in the past few weeks have seen what's behind the curtain, and there's no way to hide it anymore.

To address the increasing workload, we've been slowly building a great care team. It's been nine months since we hired Bonita, our first caregiver. She started out as occasional help, but lately, we've been increasing her hours to five or six days a week. Another addition to the team is Maria Perez, who recently started as a housekeeper, but she's jumped in and learned some caregiving skills (and, as a bonus, we get to practice our español). Now, Maureen can be gone several hours midday running errands without worry. And there is our good friend Mary who comes by every couple of weeks for my body/mind/spirit massage.

Months ago, I took on a big role for the local Walk to Defeat ALS fundraiser because they needed the help. The walk is done, and it was a great day. We were very successful in our efforts to raise money (we were the number one team). It was especially nice to have my kids and family with me, along with forty or so others. But the added work, on top of everything else I was still trying to do, took a toll on me. I said it would be my last time. Ha! I ended up being a captain for two more years, raising the most money each time. I've done my part for the Sacramento chapter of the ALS Association.

TWENTY-TWO

Prozac and Your Pecker

~

Well, maybe I lied back in November 2008, when I said I would quit writing these "ALS Updates." But I suppose it isn't really a lie if you meant it at the time. I got so many replies and such an outpouring of love and regrets, that my childhood Catholic guilt kicked in. The day after Obama's inauguration when he said, "Pick yourself up, dust yourself off, and get on with ..." I started composing this update.

Despite myself, his words inspired me. I can't bring myself to read Christopher Reeves's book or help but think Steve Hawking is insane when he said, "I can do anything I want to do." He is either delusional or has very limited aspirations. As is apparent, I am different.

It took weeks to finish this update, and as I reflect back on its evolution, I realize the stories and the tone have changed dramatically. In the beginning, they were all about travel and our adventures and coping with the realization that life *is* short.

The truth is, in November, I was down in the dumps, had been for a while, and frequently still am. So, I started taking Prozac and seeing a therapist. They both seemed to help with my depression. I had hoped the Prozac would suppress my libido since I'm stuck in this damn chair and have certain physical limitations. Maybe it's a family trait, but I'm as horny as ever. And Mr. Happy still wakes up when the situation calls for it. The only difference is, shall we say, the train takes longer to arrive at the station (not always a bad thing).

I know for a fact that doctors prescribe Prozac for treatment of premature ejaculation (there's your medical tidbit for the day). But I was in a mindset that I wanted to go and pretty soon. In fact, I did get very ill and spent two-and-a-half days in the hospital just before Christmas. I was miserable there, demanded to be sent home early, and felt like this may be it. I was ambivalent about dying right then (only because of unfinished work updating my estate plan). Three days later, we had a family Christmas party here. I barely lasted four hours. My appearance apparently shook everybody up, but I'm better now, so here we are. Unfortunately, no pill will make this go away, so maybe I should start going to marijuana bong parties with Michael Phelps.

I traditionally write these after a visit to the ALS team clinic at UCSF. We went on January 16, 2009, and it was a long, miserable day. In the end, it was hardly worth the trip. My parameters continue to plummet, and swallowing is a real problem. I'm on a pureed (baby food) diet now. Maureen puts stuff in a food processor, makes a mush, and there I go. I've reverted to infancy except for no diapers—yet. She feeds me well, and God bless her, I've only lost a little weight. At UCSF, they told us that my ability to swallow could stop within months or maybe not for years. Oh, joy! Everyone still says, "You look great!" I feel like hitting them with a stick if only I could. I know they mean well.

My arm strength remains pretty good, but my left hand is getting slow and clumsy like the right. My caregiver helps me dress and pushes me around the bathroom in a special chair from the toilet to the shower (yes, buck naked). Thankfully, I can still do my own business there.

The medicine I'd been taking for the bladder spasms stopped working, so I now wear a condom catheter with a hose to a leg bag. You never know—I could be in a conversation with you and take a piss at the same time! The *really* fun part is this: guys—picture putting a condom on your relaxed, shriveled member. It's a little tricky. Imagine your hands are useless, so the caregiver does it *for you* every morning after the shower. I know, I know—too much information.

I feel like Bernie Madoff most days when he was under house arrest. Now, of course, he is in the big house and has a cellmate named Big Dick Bubba. But lots of people visit me, and they don't have to get patted down for hacksaws or handguns. That part is nice. But, as a result, it takes me forever to get anything done because I'm always tired and take long naps. I'm like a druggie back in the 1960s—I take Valium and Vicodin at night for the leg cramps to try and sleep, and now, I'm on speed in the morning to try and stay awake. Half the time, neither works well.

So that's the update. I ran a full marathon in Humboldt in 1988, and the metaphors are apt. In retrospect, many aspects of my life trained me for what I'm going through now. My family and friends may think and pray that I have six miles to go, but I'd like to hope that I have rounded that last corner out of the redwoods and can see the finish line a hundred yards ahead.

Unfortunately, it's more likely that I have crossed that arched bridge over the stream, tearing a knee ligament in the process, and somehow, in my exhausted state, realize that I still have over a mile to go, now with a bum knee. I'm tired and anxious for the finish line. I may not be as lucky as I want to be.

At this time, I ask that people redirect their wishes and prayer focus from longevity to understanding that after almost five years, I am tired of dealing with "this bad break I caught," to quote Lou Gehrig. As I review this, the facts I've portrayed sound a bit whiny. But I don't want pity, just understanding that, despite appearances, there is not much fun left for me anymore. I have it better than most of us with ALS.

And don't blame *us* for the recession. In 2008, we bought two vehicles, paid local contractors about $25,000 to remodel the bathroom, had a painter repaint the inside of the house, hired a gardening service, and employed two part-time caregivers and a Monday through Friday housekeeper/daytime babysitter for me. All pretty much paid for with my disability income and some 401(k) money I have. I probably deserve a presidential medal or something, especially if the standard they go by is that criminal, George Tenet.

Good luck to you all who get to live through the next few years.

TWENTY-THREE

Dewey Defeats Truman

~

Here is my usual report after my visit to the UCSF-ALS Clinic on April 22, 2009. Like the last two in November and February, I felt like shit and bluntly said so. That BiPAP machine I was talking about has drastically improved my quality of life. After about six months of torture, I can sleep at night, and my nightly leg pain and bad dreams are gone.

I will digress here to answer the burning question (comparable, I'm sure, to throbbing hemorrhoids)—why will I accept BiPAP breathing assistance but refuse a feeding tube or tracheostomy? Well, reread the above paragraph—it's a quality-of-life thing, not a life-extension thing.

Although there is no miraculous cure, things are better in some ways. My symptoms keep progressing slowly. I now have more trouble swallowing and basically can't talk at all. I'm losing coordination in my *good* left hand, but at least I don't dread going to bed at night. I can stay awake most of the day and last through most conversations. I've never had that trouble for chats with family and friends since those are always interesting and thought-provoking.

My arm strength and spastic legs remain okay enough to stand for transfers, and I even can pull myself up out of my chair using the parallel bars in the bathroom. Even now, I'm actively stretching my calves, hamstrings, and back muscles twice a day while I stand there (looking down at the toilet which my caregivers usually flush if I'm nice to them). I wasn't doing that in February.

At the clinic visit, my weight was stable, my FVC breathing score actually went up again to 77 percent from 72, and my FRS function score went up a couple of points. So that should make you all happy—

until you hear that Dr. Cathy wrote on the insurance form that I was in "end-stage ALS." She finally told us—thank God—that my swallowing would go sooner than my breathing and (I think and hope) before I lose my arms.

That has been my desire all along—to stop eating and drinking and go peacefully into the arms of Morpheus via hospice. Or maybe I'll get hit by a car tomorrow! Of course, if I get bronchitis or pneumonia, I'll be outta here in a week. Anyway, who really knows?

I still have some things that I want to get done before the clock runs out, and I'm slower than molasses in February. Things like updating my will again, leaving everything to the cats, with instructions to bury me in cement under the foundation of the new Sacramento Kings Arena so I can haunt those miserable bastards for eternity.

I confused everyone who thought I was ready to die in December or January (actually, I was the person confused). Now that I seem better, everyone is going to pieces around me. Don't you just hate it when your party guest gets ready to leave, says so, and then doesn't? "Get the hook! Let me help you put on your coat!"

I'd like to express a big "Thank you!" to all who arranged, came, and worked to make the "Nachopalooza" birthday party in March a success. It was a fantastic event for my brother Tony and me. A special thanks to my daughter Carey, who worked so hard and the McGarrys.

What was I talking about? Oh, yeah, my swallowing. So I'm thinking, the way it's going and the way I cough more and more (even when I eat baby food), it probably won't be too much longer, although I've been wrong before. I won't enjoy or tolerate cream soup three times a day and can't imagine a day without coffee. Plus, I hate the cold weather, you know.

On a more serious note, two penguins walked into a bar ... (Maureen vetoed this joke, of course.) But happily, my son and his wife are expecting to make me a grandpa at the end of September. And my caregiver Leah said, "If it gets bad, couldn't you just have them put in a feeding tube so you could be there to see the baby, then have the doctor pull it out?"

Let me explain two things. As a doctor for a quarter century, I know it's difficult, if not emotionally impossible, to remove a feeding tube once it's inserted. And that would mean prolonging my progressive physical deterioration and mental suffering; so no, thank you. My mind is still here, but let's face the facts: most of "Marty Welsh" has left the premises. And second, there will always be the next thing around the corner, and sooner or later, I'll miss it. It could be the next grandkid, walking my daughter down the aisle at her marriage, or even the next blockbuster movie: *Terminator 12—The Rise of the Killer Tomatoes.*

I'll bring this to a close. If you haven't seen Craig Ferguson on *The Late Late Show* (after Letterman), record it and watch because it's excellent. And Dave Barry is still the funniest writer I have ever read, page after page. I now have a collection of his books that you may not want to borrow because there is DNA evidence of my tears, drool, and nasal contents on every other page. I've already told you about the only other orifice I empty in my chapter on curing constipation.

TWENTY-FOUR

Zachary

~

He seemed like a nice fellow, so I can't bring myself to use his real name. Or maybe I feel cautious about the libel thing. But this is the true story of a guy I'll call "Zachary" who thankfully did not kill me and gave me and my family fodder for laughs that will live through the ages.

By the time this happened, I was to the point where my legs were stiff and useless, I couldn't speak clearly and had limited use of my hands and arms (which allow me to type). More importantly, my limbs saved my life that night.

I now require paid caregivers to help me with the basics every night—getting me into my pajamas, transferring me from my wheelchair to the bed, applying the face mask, and running the BiPAP. This machine helps me to keep breathing (despite the strong sedatives to relax my muscles) through the night while I'm asleep.

In June 2009, we had a bit of a problem looming with Maureen out out of town for three days and all our regular people unavailable. So we called a service, and they recommended Zachary who, as an experienced certified nursing assistant, would have no problem.

Our first clue should've been when we interviewed him, and it turned out he did not have a CNA license. Zach appeared on time for his orientation to my routine. He seemed attentive and quite impressed with all the detailed, written, step-by-step instructions Maureen gave him. We penciled him in for three nights and two-morning shifts as well.

Zachary showed up that first night with sweat pouring off his shaved head and elsewhere (with the accompanying odor), looking tired. In fact, he said that he'd worked a lot in the last twenty-four hours.

My three brothers were visiting, so Zach and I said goodnight and proceeded to the bedroom. The fun really started while my brothers sat out on the deck, drinking scotch.

Well, it turned out Zach is deaf (we all missed seeing his hearing aids)—not a great combination with my slurred speech, not to mention the fact that he remembered *nothing* from his orientation and had the IQ of a cabbage. Oh, and his hands had a slight tremor.

With a combination of me pointing (e.g., at the toothbrush) and using my board to write directions, he managed to hook up my catheter and get me in my PJs and into bed in something over twice the usual time. By now, he probably had lost another five pounds of sweat and needed a break. Okay. He left the room for a while, used the toilet, got a glass of water, came back in, and put a bandana on his sweaty head. I wasn't too concerned since I was safe, lying on top of the bed.

At this point, wordlessly, Zachary sat down on the other bed, reading my wife's instructions. I thought, "Okay, he's just reviewing the leg range of motion exercises that come next." But after five minutes or so, he put his feet up on the bed to get comfy and continued reading. After another ten minutes (I think he was still on the same page), I finally mumbled, "Now it's time for my leg exercises."

So, I had him do just a few of these because I could feel my nighttime sedative meds kicking in, and I needed the BiPAP pretty quickly. I then watched with some apprehension as he tried to figure out how to assemble the parts. I ended up putting the head strap on by myself since he couldn't figure it out. He put the mask on and, after a bit of fumbling, managed to turn on the airflow.

The trick with this thing is to keep the air leakage around my nose and mouth to a minimum. Between twenty-two and twenty-five is a good range for minimal leakage. Much more than that, I can feel it, and you can hear it. The machine's alarm is set to go off at fifty because: 1) I frequently get up during the night which results in much higher numbers and 2) the alarm is loud and obnoxious for Maureen and me.

Zach started it, and I felt it leaking like crazy from both sides. I guessed it wouldn't be good, so I wrote a note, "What's the leak number?"

He looked at the machine and said, "Four point zero." At this point, I was screwed anyway, so I fiddled with the nostril pieces myself with my (better) left hand and waved Zachary off to bed. *Qué será, será.* Then (I didn't see him do this), he took his hearing aids out and went right to sleep.

Amazingly, I slept through until 2:30 a.m. That's when the real fun started. The left nostril piece blew clean out, and with my deviated septum and a bit of nasal congestion on the right, I couldn't breathe. That woke me up. Asphyxiation will do that. With my left hand, I pried the mask away from my face (fighting the elastic straps) so I could breathe. Because the leak was now huge, I waited for the alarm to go off, and sure enough, it did.

Beep, beep! ... Beep, beep!

And all I heard was Zachary snoring in his bed two feet away. And more snoring.

Beep, beep! ... Beep, beep! This noise went on for about a minute.

I managed to get my dysfunctional, weaker right hand up to my face, using it to pry the mask away so I could breathe. With my left hand, I grabbed the bell we left on the bedside table and started ringing it.

Ring, ring! ... Beep, beep! ... Ring, ring! ... Beep, beep!

More snoring.

So I started banging the bell on the table as I rang it, still prying the mask away with my weak right hand to still breathe. The air leak sounded like a Category 2 hurricane. It must have been a pretty funny sight. Too bad Zach missed it.

But he finally woke up! He slowly sat up, yawned, stretched, sat on the end of my wife's bed, looked at me and said, "Hi, what's up?"

I'll quickly end the misery here by saying he immediately figured out that something was wrong with the mask which he reapplied (again with a big leak, but I handled it), then he went back to his bed and was soon snoring again.

I laid there for twenty minutes or so, very grateful I hadn't died a horrible death of asphyxiation while figuring out how to handle the next two nights and days. I was firing Zach first thing in the morning, of course, and the schedule had nothing but his name for all of those shifts. I finally fell asleep.

As he got me out of bed in the morning, I had one of my brothers set me up with the computer that I now use to speak. I took Zachary in the back bedroom and (quite politely, considering) sacked Zach.

Luckily, I did this before telling my brothers. In fact, they knew something was going on when Zach walked out the door with all his stuff (he was scheduled for three days). They were bugging me to tell them what was going on.

I wisely waited until he drove off to tell them. After they stopped laughing and it sunk in what might have happened (i.e., dead Marty), they got a bit upset (as we Irish can do) and would've gone and beat the shit out of him.

So that's it for Zach. I'm lucky my family was here because we all pulled together and got someone for the nights. The next morning, after a crash course, one of my brothers was a better help than the next guy from the agency. Of course, when Maureen called to check in, we had the set of lies ready, "Everything's fine!"

Here are a few sample emails that have been pouring in from my brothers since then:

From Tony:

"Oh, Zach, we would like to say, 'So long!'
Put on your damn hearing aids!
The alarm didn't wake you,
The cowbell didn't shake you,
Rule Boy couldn't break you,
So unemployment will have to take you!"

From Greg:

"I'm beat; I'm going to lie down and take a Zachary."
"Man, I slept like a Zachary last night!"
"Zach and Zacharier."
"I'm Irish, and I've got a hankering for some corned beef and Zachary."
"My favorite side dish with BBQ is Zachary slaw."
A horror film title: *Bedtime with Zachary*

From David:
"Hey, guys! Zachary left his favorite compilation CD behind."
"Cold Sweat"—Stevie Ray Vaughn
"I'm So Tired"—The Beatles
"Dream a Little Dream"—The Mamas and the Papas
"Tommy, Can You Hear Me?"—The Who
"Hello, It's Me"—Todd Rundgren
"Get Up, Stand Up"—Bob Marley
"I Wanna Be Sedated"—The Ramones
"I'll Be Seeing You"—Frank Sinatra
"Hit the Road, Jack"—Ray Charles

So, that's the story of "Zachary."

TWENTY-FIVE

Top Ten Signs You're Looking at a Bad Caregiver

~

Your caregiver:

1. has the IQ of your typical vegetable.
2. has the personality of cheap lawn furniture.
3. is deaf and can't hear the alarm—which means you're about to die.
4. shows up on a motorcycle wearing jeans, a t-shirt, and a baseball cap on backward and reeking of cigarettes.
5. is billed as a CNA, but is still working on it.
6. has a skull and crossbones tattoo—anywhere.
7. wants to be paid under the table (i.e., wants you to participate in their income tax fraud).
8. insists on doing things their way even when you tell them what works best for you.
9. has to be reminded how to do something not once, not twice, but three times (see #1).
10. There is no ten—if you haven't figured it out by now, you have the IQ of a typical vegetable and deserve them.

TWENTY-SIX

Sex, Drugs, and Rock 'n' Roll

I'm sure you're thinking, "What the heck is a guy with advanced ALS doing writing an article with a title like that? Is he demented?" Well, yes, I am, but that's not the point. The point is when you're given a diagnosis like this, or terminal cancer, or your pecker is about to turn green and fall off, I believe most people don't crawl into a hole forever. It's a rude shock to be sure. But after a time, you focus more on things in general and some in particular.

And if you think I'm going to be discussing my sex life with my wife here, you're crazy. Maureen is always so helpful with editing all this nonsense I put on paper, and she'd *never* let me have any discussion about our sex life. So, forget it. Probably.

That said, this chapter is still PG-13 or maybe even R rated—we'll have to see what comes out of my deranged mind. You parents don't want to be reading this in front of your kids because you would have some explaining to do (about your snickering).

I thought up this topic and title a while ago after talking with my morning caregiver Jessica. We were discussing how she had taken her two teenage sons in for "the talk" with their doctor. You know, the talk about sex, the dangers of drugs, and how cool rock 'n' roll is (I know the guy, and he loves it).

Jessica is younger than us, on the good side of forty, and is now a fixture in our home in the mornings. At this point, Maureen and I consider her a friend as much as anything, and we discuss all kinds of things. And she is, well, cute. But that's just a fact, like saying Maureen is cute, so I don't think Maureen will edit it out. Jessica is married to a wonderful guy (which is how I feel about Maureen, as you know), and they have four boys between them! Keep this in mind for later.

Let's go backward and start with rock 'n' roll. I love all kinds of music, so back in 2008, we made a real push to get out and hear some live. Even though I was already in the wheelchair, I still had the stamina. If you'll recall from earlier updates, we went to listen to Big Band Swing and Zydeco at the Sacramento Jazz Festival. We saw Wayman Tisdale (smooth, pop jazz) at the Radisson (where Tina made her appearance). We bought tickets for the Dave Matthews Band, but because of the untimely death of his sax player, LeRoi Moore, they canceled the show.

Then, last summer, we went up to Lake Tahoe to see James Taylor and his band for the *Covers* tour. It was a great show and also my last night away from home. Even in a handicap hotel room, it just doesn't work anymore.

Early last fall, the best and last happened when we learned that the band Journey, with new Filipino singer Arnel Pineda, was doing a show in Sacramento. (By the way, whether you like Journey or not, they have a great story about how they found Pineda to replace Steve Perry.) We got great seats near the front and thought we'd go for it, even if it meant getting home at midnight (energy-wise, I usually crash about nine).

Of course, this leads to the next topic: drugs. I have pretty intense muscle spasms with my ALS, so I have to take enough muscle relaxers to put down a charging rhino. I'm habituated to them now, so I can stay awake during the day with two cups of coffee and Ritalin (a.k.a. speed), which I take every morning. I'm basically a junkie.

Naturally, I was worried I'd be sleepy during the show which didn't start until after eight. Hmm, what to do? Aha! I'll pop some extra uppers! It'll be just like the old days, back in the 1970s. But wait a minute—I never *did* that (I was a nerdy pre-med. Honest, kids). I only smoked some weed in college. (Who didn't back then?) *And* I inhaled because as someone famously said recently, "That was the point!" The stuff back then just kinda made me mellow and say, "Groovy" and "I dig it, man" a lot. That, and eating an extra-large pizza by myself at three in the morning along with some M&Ms I found under the couch cushion.

But at this juncture in my life, I thought, "What the hell, I'll try drugs to keep me awake." So, I took one or two just outside the gates as we went in. Well, the concert was fantastic. Pineda not only sounds identical to Perry but has become a world-class front man, and I stayed awake for the show and the drive home! Of course, in retrospect, I think a cup or two of coffee would've had the same effect.

So my point is—what the heck was I talking about? Oh yeah, drugs. They fry your brain, kids! So instead of speed, take triple shot espressos, and instead of Valium or marijuana, go ahead and have that third martini with lunch. It's okay! It must be because our government says so (even if they imposed Prohibition back in the 1920s, then repealed it because it was a total failure). What does history matter to an advanced society like ours? The End!

Haha! Not really! Here's the part I added *after* Maureen did her editing. The part about S-E-X! You *know* you wanted it, so here goes: what's good about ALS is it doesn't affect the area just south of the Mason-Dixon Line, if you get my drift. But once you lose your legs (I've been in a wheelchair almost two years now), a couple of things happen.

I never was the Brad Pitt of my generation, but since when does a guy's equipment even know or care about that? Being in a wheelchair and unable to talk is an undeniable blow to your self-image as Clark Gable reincarnated. Plus, without the use of your legs, there are certain technical difficulties with, we will use the fencing terms, *thrust and parry.* So, you have to get creative, and I'll leave it at that.

A man isn't meant to sit in a wheelchair all day long, every day, and not have some deleterious effects. One big problem is that my muscles have started to shrivel up, although my weight is relatively stable (crucial with ALS) since Maureen is great at making delicious meals for me. Unfortunately, that means *my body is turning to fat!*

I've watched my belly grow such that my navel now looks like the proverbial hole dug to China. And as I look down at my thighs while sitting on the pot (remember that these same thighs got me through a marathon once), I'm reminded of two beached albino elephant seals. All of which adds up to this: I now resemble Jabba the Hutt from *Star Wars.*

Except that he had Princess Leia on a chain in a bikini. Are there any volunteers out there?

Most mornings, you'll find me sitting on the can, surrounded by my rolls of blubber, reading Dave Barry. He makes me laugh so hard that the toilet bowl becomes like a cosmic black hole with infinite gravitational suction. I have to hold onto my tonsils to keep them from exiting. Then, I put down the book and say, "Whoa!" That's because I occasionally look down and notice that I look like an uncircumcised chipmunk. ("Did it get sucked down the toilet?") Fortunately, no. He's still there—just hiding in the rolls while my entire mind focuses on not falling off the seat from laughing.

There's a trick question asked in med school anatomy class: "What organ of the male body can grow more than ten times in size?" Once everyone in the lecture hall stops squirming and the girls stop giggling, the professor says, "Why, the pupil, of course." From one millimeter in bright light to ten millimeters in the dark, for you nerds out there.

Well, I beg to differ about the answer to that trick question, at least in my case, but I digress. You unmarried ladies out there probably don't fully see this, but Mr. Presto Change-O can alter his appearance for the better in a matter of seconds. Going the other way takes longer, but you single gals only see the captain in full military position (I would hope).

Sorry for the medical/anatomical digression. Although with ALS, thank God, it's not a complete *use-it-or-lose-it* scenario. I'm a doctor and have seen thousands of tallywhackers. The boys in the duffel bag are not large for my size, but they apparently work overtime and never take a vacation.

And the master of ceremonies is, under the proper circumstances, only slightly above average. My wife has to buy the large size condom catheters for me, but gosh sakes, I'm six feet four. Sorry girls, sometimes big feet just means you have to buy big shoes.

Anyway, although I'm tall, I would've been laughed off the set of some of those movies I've accidentally rented in hotel rooms. I mean, come on! Is there a mad scientist out there cloning male humans with horses? Where do they get some of these guys? But if you're over twenty-five and haven't yet realized that a guy's biggest sexual organ is—his brain, then you have my deepest sympathies. At least, your wife or girlfriend does. I'm sure I'm not the only guy out there who has done his duty two or three times, only to be awakened at four in the morning by the girl next to you saying, "Wake up, sailor. I need some more of *that*!"

Where was I? Oh, yeah, wheezer and the twins. Now here I am in my life where the thoroughly professional (and as I said earlier, cute) Jessica has to wheel me around naked into the shower, washing my hair and armpits since I can't raise my arms over shoulder level anymore. That is a psychological hurdle for me (one of many) that I knew was coming for years and still dreaded. But you get over it. Still, I'm careful not to look at her or make eye contact. And, occasionally, I either do math problems in my head or think of my grandmother's eighty-year-old Hungarian landlady who always wore black (including her knee-high nylons that drooped around her ankles).

Fortunately, my arms and hands still allow me to soap and wash off Mr. Happy and the backup band, so Jessica leaves me alone to do that. But even then, with me doing the washing, he starts to wake up and says, "Hullo, Guv. Is it teatime? Any crumpets about?" Fortunately, washing that part of your anatomy takes a short time, and he's back snoozing when it's time to be toweled off.

What I'm getting to is this—I sincerely hope I'm dead before I can no longer do that particular job. I definitely don't want Jessica to do this because—like a good three-point shooter in basketball—the drill sergeant has no memory and no conscience. And *that* would be embarrassing.

I guess the answer is—this chapter is rated "R."

Twenty-Seven

This Just In

~

Here we go again. I'd never have guessed five years ago that I'd still be writing the "ALS Updates." On July 15, 2009, we went to the UCSF-ALS Clinic, and I am duty-bound to tell you that I'm still warming the globe, just to spite Al Gore.

We had another easy day of it on Wednesday. Up at 6:00 a.m., left at 9:30, no traffic, in the clinic for three hours, and home by 5:30 p.m. Every three months is about all we can handle of that, and it's a vast improvement over the Friday team clinic slog which usually lasted thirteen to fifteen hours.

Sgt. Joe Friday is peering over my shoulder, so here are the facts. They think I'm doing well. My weight only dropped two pounds because Maureen feeds me so well. My FVC breathing score dropped a bit from 77 percent to 70, although my diaphragm force is still pegging at the top of the needle. My appetite and swallowing are about the same. Since my speech is mostly unintelligible, I use the computer to talk for me more often. Thankfully, I can still hunt-and-peck with my index fingers and left thumb.

Well, I'm slowly but surely getting weaker everywhere, most noticeably in my arms and quads. Since last April, I can no longer pull myself up to standing position without a little push. I still stand for transfers and stretches twice a day, and that feels *really* good. With my quads going and my hamstrings and back muscles still strong and tight, I work every day to keep them stretched out so I can stand. It's all about prevention. I have paid caregivers every day now, except in emergencies when Maureen has to fill in. Our housekeeper Maria is here with me during most weekdays so Maureen can go to the store, etc. Of course, this is all quite costly which is why I'm fortunate to have sufficient disability insurance and my 401(k) if needed. I don't have long-term care insurance, but Maureen does now after seeing what can happen. That's why I'm supporting the ALS Association and Partners In Care (a local group) to provide funds for people who need this help and aren't as fortunate as me.

Last month, poor Maureen lost her mother Pat, just a year after her dad died, but after fifty-nine years of marriage, it's a familiar story. Pat's health was up and down during the last year. She even made a trip up here to visit. In the end, it happened over the course of one week. Thankfully, the family was able to be there which was good. Except me, of course—I can no longer sleep anywhere but here.

What else? We had a Welsh family reunion of sorts up here one weekend when Maureen was down in King City, attending to family business. I was expecting my brother Greg on Friday, but when we returned from a quick trip to town, there were my other two brothers waiting to surprise me as well. And they did! The four of us had a great evening. It was lucky they were here because that was the weekend we had the crisis with the incompetent caregiver Zach who is now part of the family lore.

Most days, I remain pretty busy for four hours or so, working on the computer, making some DVDs, writing, and getting out a few times a week to go to a movie, an appointment, or shopping. But things sap my energy fairly quickly now, so I need to pace myself or pay the price. I watch a lot of DVDs on TV, and I keep my mental to-do list always full and beyond what I can accomplish, so that keeps me going. Mostly.

Oh, and this just in—an essay I wrote was published in the *Los Angeles Times's* Sunday Op-Ed section (July 26, 2009) entitled "100 Things Leading to a Single Choice." It's about quality-of-life issues, end-of-life decisions, and the slippery slopes that are out there. This article is my fifteen minutes of fame, thanks to my sister Melinda. That's about it for now. The Sacramento ALS Walk Fundraiser is Saturday, October 17. To my surprise, it's looking like the 2008 walk won't be my last one.

TWENTY-EIGHT

100 Things Leading to a Single Choice

~

This chapter originated as an Op-Ed in the Los Angeles Times *in 2009.*

As his health fades, a doctor's acceptance of death over excessive medical intervention illuminates the difference between life and living.

Martin Welsh grew up in Los Angeles and graduated from UCLA Medical School. He now resides with his wife in Camino, California.

I'm a fifty-five-year-old retired family doctor with a large, loving family, innumerable friends, and former patients whom I see often. I'm an extraordinarily lucky man. For the last five years, I have also been a patient. I have ALS (or Lou Gehrig's disease), a cruel neurological illness where a normally functioning intellect becomes trapped in an increasingly weak and eventually paralyzed body. Soon, I will die from it.

Throughout my career, I tried to honor my patients' end-of-life wishes. But after a quarter century as a firsthand witness to death, I've developed my own perspective. It's not that I'm a quitter. I've struggled against adversity of one sort or another all my life, and those challenges have helped prepare me for what I face now. I still delight in accomplishing difficult things, and I always wear a bright red ALS wristband that says, "Never Give Up."

That said, there will come a limit. I have made it very clear to my wife, my family, and my doctors that I want no therapy that will prolong my suffering and lengthen the burden on others. I do not want a feeding tube nor a tracheostomy when the time comes that I can no longer eat, drink, or even breathe for myself.

Physicians and families sometimes feel an obligation to do all that can be done to keep someone alive. I believe this is based in equal measure on a fear of death and on Western medicine's increasing ability to prolong life near its end. I was able to diagnose myself at a fairly early stage of the disease. My case was slower to progress than some, and so I was able to keep working as a physician for nearly two years. During that time, I was enormously grateful—for my patients, for sunsets, for golf games with good friends. Life has been truly wonderful, even as I have slowly lost the use of my hand, then an arm, then both legs, and my speech.

As much as I have stayed focused on what I'm still able to do, it has become harder to ignore the things I'm losing. Today, my guitars sit idle, and I haven't used my stethoscope in years. My jogging shoes gather dust in a closet as I watch my belly grow from lack of exercise. I remember the last time I tried to shoot a free throw with a basketball, and I was five feet short of the rim.

Today, I find myself facing the kind of quality-of-life issues I discussed innumerable times with my patients. Answers vary from person to person. But the fundamental question is always this: At what point is quality of life no longer worth the emotional and physical costs of maintaining it?

I am not afraid of dying or death, and that is a wonderfully comforting thing for me right now. As a physician, I have seen so many *good* deaths in my time, so I know this passage can be peaceful, spiritual, and even comforting to those left behind. I hope for such a death.

I've also started to think about how I'll know when I am ready for it. To that end, I often think about what I call the "100 Things." Here's how it works. Imagine a list of 100 things you do most days. Some are routine, some are chores, and some are pleasurable. Get out of bed and walk to the bathroom. Kiss your wife. Answer the phone. Drive your car to work. Play golf with your friends. Brush your teeth. Write a letter, lick and seal the envelope closed, and put a stamp on it. Hug your child.

Of course, we do much more than 100 things each day, but for now, just imagine 100 that are essential to the life you live. If you take one away, you can still do ninety-nine. Is life worth living without being able to smell the rose in the garden? Of course, it is! How about losing two or seven, or twenty-three—is life still worth living? Of course.

But suppose you get to where you've lost, say, ninety things, and now with each thing taken away, a bad thing is added. You can no longer walk well, you start falling, and it hurts. Your grip is gone, and you also suffer the ignominy of wetting your pants because of bladder spasms. You can't turn over in bed, and that also means you will get bedsores unless someone turns you frequently. Life is still worth living, but you're getting tired.

At some point, no matter who you are or how strong, you can lose enough things that matter—and acquire enough negatives—that the burdens will outweigh the joys of being alive. This is the stage when, as a doctor, I'd reassure my patients and their families that they had fought the good fight, and it was now okay to accept moving to the next phase.

I know that one day I will reach that point, which is why I worry about feeding tubes and ventilators. It's been my experience that there are times where these things start almost automatically, and once they start, they are next to impossible to stop.

I've seen too many unfortunate people kept alive for years in hospitals or nursing homes, beyond all quality of life. Sometimes it causes untold stress in a family. Some of these cases even have made national news, and, unbelievably, our government and some national religious leaders even weighed in—as if they had a right to do so.

I worry that, at some point, a feeding tube or another artificial substitute for a basic body function will be medically *indicated* in my case. Intervention at that time might seem to make sense to those around me. But the result may be that I am kept alive only to count off the remaining things on my list of 100, such that I'm forced to live well past where I would want to say, "Enough."

I like to know where a road leads before I set out on a journey. Right now, one path I could take leads to a place I do not want to go. I am determined not to start down that path, even if others think I'm premature in my decision. In short, I may well be ready to die before my family and friends are ready to say goodbye. But they know that, as I face my diminishing list of 100 things that make life worth living—the choice of quality over quantity has to be mine to make.

This article was also featured as the narrative for Marty's appearance in the documentary Consider the Conversation.

TWENTY-NINE

Shit Happens

~

From an early age, we all intuitively know that shit happens. Some of us even do it when we're in the delivery room, fresh out of the oven, and it's okay (if this happens, your mom might need a C-section). But later on in childhood, we find out that bad things just come into our lives. And usually in threes. Why that is, no scientist has ever been able to explain. It would be worthy of a Nobel Prize. But we all know it's true. Except when it's not, like the month I just had.

It started as a typical day, although it had been a long and intense week with a lot of visitors, so I was worn down. Anyway, that night as I went to bed, my abdomen gurgled. Then another gurgle, and I thought to myself, "Oh my God, I'm about to have diarrhea!"

I frantically rang the bell for Maureen, and then it was like the final scenes of *Animal House*—where chaos reigned and people ran around Main Street in their underwear with their hair on fire. I panicked. Maureen tried to get me and my spastic legs out of bed, into the wheelchair, to the bathroom, on the commode chair, over the drop zone—and we didn't make it.

I left shit all over the bathroom floor. And I mean, *all over* the floor. I saw traces of food I ate a week ago. And the areas I missed, Maureen's feet took care of since she unavoidably stepped in it and spread it around. It felt like some of my stomach lining may have ended up on the tile. After that, of course, it was a hazmat cleanup job for my wife, a shower for me, etc. Not so funny at midnight. But that was just the start.

Over the course of the next two weeks, my power wheelchair broke down—with 200-plus-pound me in the fully reclined position.

I was dead weight, lifted out of the chair, courtesy of Leah, the strongest of my caregivers. I still don't know how she did it.

Later on, my power recliner in the living room broke down with me in—you guessed it—the reclined position. Of course, the battery was dead on the Hoyer Lift that could've pulled me out of the chair. Three separate times, our caregivers (who are crucial to my care while Maureen is out working) had their cars break down or called in sick at the last minute. I felt like Job from the Bible. Meanwhile, Maureen was about to shoot someone. There was bad juju hovering over the house like a cloud. Dogs and cats were sleeping together due to raining scorpions. The rule of threes was out the window. Several other things happened that, mercifully, I have forgotten. So I reacted the way any normal person would under the circumstances, especially with the whole progressing ALS thing in the background. I finally broke down and cried like a little girl.

No. Of course, I'm lying (if you believe that, you weren't paying attention). I had Jessica paint my toenails in flames (for August) and do my hair in a Mohawk. It was the only sensible way to respond.

THIRTY

I Haven't Died Yet

~

Well, it seems I haven't died yet. I'm like the weird neighbor down the street who keeps saying he's leaving the dinner party. Although an hour later, he's still guzzling your wine and eating what was going to be leftovers for tomorrow's dinner.

We went to the UCSF-ALS Clinic again on Wednesday, October 21, 2009. So here, as usual, is my report on how I'm doing and what's happening. Hard to believe, but this is my sixteenth "ALS Update." I diagnosed myself over five years ago on May 28, 2004, but it took a while for me to convince other experts that a small-town country doc knew what he had. So here's what happened at the clinic. I'm losing my quads and upper arms now and need a big push to stand and bear weight for transfers (seven times a day). My FVC breathing score dropped from 70 percent to 60. To my dismay, I gained weight, although everyone else is happy, as usual. Dr. Cathy says you typically lose one pound of muscle a month, so that means (subtract the nine and carry the one) I must have put on about ten pounds of fat these last three months! Eskimos with harpoons will be waiting outside to harvest my blubber!

Since breathing is essential, the respiratory therapist at the ALS Clinic increased the settings on my nighttime BiPAP breathing assist to help expand my lungs more. I'm trying to be more diligent about my breathing exercises, and I don't care what they say—I'm going to stop eating dessert every night. I said to the clinic team, "See you in January."

I'm definitely physically weakening, and some days are worse than others. It depends a lot on my mood, and how well I've slept. Unlike three months ago, I can't do stretching exercises for my calves and back.

We received the Hoyer Lift for transfers in December 2008, when I almost died and was weak for days. Although we kept it for emergencies, I'm afraid that, soon, I'll be using it routinely. I'm resisting it so far, but I want to start using it before I fall and split my head open.

My ability to swallow is decreasing. I can't drink water, OJ, or clear juice anymore. The thickening agent is awful, so now my liquid intake is nectar, smoothies, or soup. For some reason, I still manage coffee, thank God. I need it to stay awake from 11:30 a.m. to 3:00 p.m.—the limit of my stamina for typing or doing anything except napping and watching TV.

Emotionally, I've always had up-and-down days, although lately, they seem a bit more frequent. I'm pretty sure I have that particular type of emotional dementia that most people with ALS get called the "Pseudo-Bulbar Affect." Supposedly, it makes some people laugh or cry inappropriately. Fortunately, I have the former. There's a drug to even you out, but they've stopped asking me if I want it because my reply is always, "Are you nuts?"

So when Jessica combs my hair, or Leah does my range-of-motion leg exercises, I start laughing because I suddenly remember a part of Wanda Sykes's *HBO Comedy Special*. What could be better than that?

I *really* need to retire. I can't keep up this pace; it's exhausting, and I get grouchy. In early 2006, I was working part-time and thinking that I'd be waking up and the big decision for the day would be whether or not to polish my shoes.

Since my last "ALS Update" in July, I have:

- had my "100 Things" article published in the *Los Angeles Times*. http://articles.latimes.com/2009/jul/26/opinion/oe-welsh 26 Without my sister Melinda's help, this article would not have happened. It was reprinted all over the country, in Canada, and translated into Mandarin for a So Cal Chinese radio station;
- responded to many of the hundreds of grateful letters and emails about the article;
- been filmed for a documentary that should air on PBS in late 2010;

- been the leading individual fundraiser for the October Sacramento ALS Walk;
- had a front-page "Above the Fold" article about me published in the *Sacramento Bee:* http://www.sacbee.com/296/story/2183064.html?storylink=lingospot_related_articles;
- been trying to finish up the last parts of my book which I foresee as being a challenge to publish since I won't be available for a book signing tour;
- been trying to do my usual daily tasks like fixing the computer network crash I just caused at our home office.

Shit. So much for imagining myself sitting back and watching sports and movies on TV.

The highlight of the summer was Labor Day weekend when Terry Kaldhusdal and Mike Bernhagen flew out from Wisconsin to film me for part of their documentary on end-of-life issues.

This is Terry's fifth documentary, and he knows what he's doing. He's already sent us a first cut nine-minute piece on my part, and it's wowed everyone who has seen it.

We capped off Saturday evening with a dinner party for twenty-seven on the deck, spectacularly catered by Mike, my caregiver Jessica's husband. I pooped out at nine, thanked everyone, and said I wanted the party to go on, even though I had to go off to bed with Tarah (my cute blonde twenty-seven-year-old caregiver). That brought the house down and was a great way to end the day. (A guy can dream, can't he?)

I became a grandpa on September 27, when Kevin's wife Kristen gave birth to Alexis Emily Welsh in Phoenix. I'm looking forward to seeing them all during Thanksgiving week. And I've had lovely visits from my daughter Carey, and all five of my siblings. I cherish all these times and memories.

Oh, and I can't forget my lovely wife Maureen, who keeps the house running efficiently and peacefully while I sit on my arse, typing nonsense like this and making life difficult. I'll end on that note. This chapter is already longer than most. Maybe I'll write another in January; maybe I'll catch pneumonia instead. Either way, I've had a great run, better than most, and every day is a new adventure.

THIRTY-ONE

Whazzup with the Toenails?

~

If you're reading this, it means the publisher has completely lost his or her mind and printed this with color photographs. So, I need to explain the toenail art.

In February of 2009, Vickie Sugich and Mary Walden, two of my whacko friends, babysat me. By then, I'd been in a wheelchair for over a year, so they decided it would be hilarious to paint my toenails red for Valentine's Day.

As Vickie painted them, she said, "Don't move right now. I'm doing a smiley face on your big toe."

To which I replied (in my garbled voice), "I *can't* move my legs—that's why I'm in the f**king wheelchair!"

Everyone laughed when they saw my toes—not with me, but *at* me—something I've been accustomed to all my life. So in March, for Saint Patrick's Day, they insisted on redoing them in green. Since I'm of Irish ancestry (75 percent), I couldn't refuse *that.*

Several months later, Jessica, my morning caregiver, came on board the team. It turns out Jessica is a caregiver in the mornings and a hair stylist/cosmetologist in the afternoons. This arrangement works out great since she cuts my hair and does my fingernails and toenails when they need it.

When she saw pictures of two previous tortures, she had to get in on the act, of course. By then, I had given up any sense of self-dignity or manliness, and so I just said, "I am your canvas, do what you want." Now, every month, whether I need it or not, I get a new paint job after she trims my nails.

My brothers think I've been in the closet all these years and am now *outed.* As for me, what do I care anymore? It makes people laugh and think I'm nuts (which I am). As I write this (February 2010), I think I'll be dead soon, anyway. So that's the story.

THIRTY-TWO

Too Much Information

~

I use this chapter title to honor one of my brothers (he shall remain anonymous) who said exactly that. (You know who you are, Greg.)

By the summer of 2009, I had worn a condom catheter for a year or more since the meds no longer stopped my bladder spasms. Not to mention the fact that I couldn't wheel into a bathroom and stand up even briefly to use a urinal or even hold on to what was always leaky, damp plumbing.

So these condom caths (a.k.a. rubbers with a hole at the end) aren't lubricated for your pleasure as the other kind are. In fact, quite the opposite. They have mild adhesive on the inside to keep them from slipping off. But the result is, when you change them every day for your shower, they pull your hairs down there! I know—TMI.

Ouch! I'm not like the hairy, gorilla guys you see walking around. I have an average rug down there, so I started shaving. The result was not like what girls do: landing strip, bikini triangle, or anything like that. The result was purely functional and looked like one of those aerial photos from Britain of an alien crop circle—except for a deformed one-eyed Easter Island head in the middle. Sorry for the visual, but facts are facts.

All was fine until my hands got bad enough that I thought, "Do I really want a sharp razor blade down next to my privates when, at any moment, I could slip or start clonus in my hand?" (Clonus is a violent, uncontrollable shaking I get with my ALS.) The answer became "No" when I nicked the master sergeant one morning. I told Jessica that next time, it was now her job. She didn't react other than, "I'm glad you didn't cut it off before you finally asked me. I've been waiting."

So, being "Rule Boy," I wrote her up some directions as follows.

Jessica:

I know you told me that you experimented with your husband Mike (I'm sure Dr. Oz hopes that led to some fun and games, or maybe you guys are worse off than I imagined), but here are my thoughts.

How to Shave My Wee Pecker

(At least, I hope he behaves and stays that way.)

1. Remember this: You can yank on the frank but handle the beans *gently!*
2. The hair down there is for God knows what evolutionary purpose, but it hurts to pull off the condom catheter when it's overgrown. It only needs shaving *where it gets in the way! No Brazilian shit!*
3. Take it all off the shaft. You can yank on the frank for traction and shave downward—*away* from the operational end.
4. Shave around the base of the shaft as much and as far away as needed so that no long buggers catch in the damn catheter glue.
5. You may need to shave some on my lower abdomen and upper thighs, but for God's sake, don't get carried away.
6. If the beans in the duffle bag need lifting, try pulling upward with one finger, right in the middle (anatomically, the median raphe). Another way is to lift the whole thing up gently—not like a baggage handler at the airport.

That is your medical lesson for today. You're welcome. Co-signed by the big head and the little one, both named "Marty." On second thought, maybe Greg was right after all.

THIRTY-THREE

Yankie the Wankie

~

I said I might get pneumonia last October, but I didn't. We were back in San Francisco at the ALS Clinic on January 6, 2010.

This "ALS Update" will be the last in my book. It may seem stark, but at this point, it's an honest portrayal of my life. Typing is getting increasingly hard, and it's time to finish the book and start the process of trying to get it published. In April, maybe there will be another one; maybe I'll do it; maybe Maureen will send one out for me; maybe I'll be harpooned by the Eskimos for my blubber. Who knows? I sure don't.

It's been an eventful three months. The best way to summarize is this—I hate Decembers. In 2007, we pushed the schedule so hard that we collapsed for two weeks in January which prompted me to revise one of "The ALS Rules" from "Push my limits" to "Pace myself (and Maureen)."

In December 2008, I came down with a urinary tract infection and was nearly septic, could have died from a resistant bacterial infection, spent two miserable days in the hospital, and came home against medical advice. I consciously chose to go on living for a while, at least.

Last month, we thought we had spaced out our activities. But last week, I still got sick. I was so stressed out that I made one of the most regrettable decisions of my life and am only now beginning to feel rested again. I'm hoping for no more repeat Decembers, but I'm a notoriously terrible prognosticator. So again, who knows? It's not up to me.

The clinic trip was surprisingly short—we left at 10:00 a.m. and got home at 5:15. There was no traffic, and we had a shorter visit because the respiratory therapist was absent. There were no stops on the way down—just a caffeine drive-by on the way home. Although I was curious to see what my FVC breathing score was (it had dropped precipitously last time), we felt good about going because we got some great advice from Dr. Cathy and others during our brief visit.

Really, what difference would it make knowing my FVC score? I already use the BiPAP machine all night. I also use it for my two daytime naps. Without its help, I'm told that my lips turn blue when I'm asleep (generally not a good sign). And I'm getting short of breath with very minimal effort.

I'll digress a minute since they asked me to relay a plug to all of you in California to check off that little box near the top of your state tax return and give some of your refund—if only five to ten dollars—to ALS research. Last year (also the first year), it raised $200,000. Unless $250,000 is raised in one year (within the first two years), they take the ALS Association off the form.

I was irritated because, once again, I *gained* weight (five pounds). I still have a good appetite and eat whatever is in front of me. I was raised that way as you of my generation know. ("You owe it to the starving pagan babies in Africa.") What total bullshit, but we had to clean our plates. So, I blame my weight gain on Maureen. I apologize to my fellow PALS (People with ALS) who are predictably losing weight.

My functional rating score has now dropped to seventeen (out of forty). With a big push in the morning, I can still stand up (barely). Another task involves holding on to the bars when getting on or off the toilet/shower chair and pulling up my pants. Other than these, I'm a rag doll. I have to let someone shower me, shave me, and get me dressed without my help at all. I use the Hoyer Lift to transfer from chair to bed at night because by then, my legs cannot be trusted to bear any weight.

I now have one of those special spoons with an adaptive grip. Lately, I've started to allow someone feed me when my arms are too tired, which is nearly every evening. I'm still able to type, use the TV remote, and work the hospital bed controls with my left hand and fingers. I can raise a half-full plastic cup to my mouth, although it feels like a hundred pounds. Not for long though. I've just started using a straw occasionally.

Swallowing has become more difficult. I routinely cough when I eat or drink because some little thing sticks in my windpipe (but no major panic attacks yet). My upper arm strength is comparable to my three-month-old granddaughter's. I rest my elbows as much as possible on the chair arms to eat or type. I haven't read a newspaper in months, and it's even become difficult to pick up small paperbacks and turn the pages. So goes the progression to complete paralysis.

My day starts at 4:30 a.m. when Maureen's alarm goes off. It's her reminder to give me a muscle relaxer so that I can bend my legs. Then, after a little more sleep, I get out of bed. I watch the light come through the south-facing windows while I have coffee. Out of habit, I think of a list of things I want to do that day, knowing now that I'll be lucky to get half of them done. The caregiver arrives at 7:30 a.m. I start a three-to-four-hour routine that leaves me exhausted and in need of a two-hour nap.

I hit the computer around one, answer emails, and put the final touches on the pieces that I hope to form into a book. After three hours or so, I'm done for and off to sleep again for two more hours. I wake up, have dinner, and for a few hours, watch The *PBS News Hour* or a movie or something. Then, the p.m. caregiver arrives at eight-thirty, and I'm off to bed.

That's it, day in and day out, seven days a week. We rarely go out to a movie or cruise around the block or have a visitor. If we do, I'm completely worthless the next day. I'm a sad sack of shit at this point. I can't think of any new ways to reinvent myself. I've gone from doctor/athlete/musician to DVD producer/emailer/book writer. And now, I'm close to becoming a piece of beloved furniture.

This will be hard to take for very long, but ultimately, it isn't up to me. As I've said before, I don't believe in suicide, assisted or not, or euthanasia. However, I do believe that it's my right to refuse a feeding tube or ventilator, as I said in my *Los Angeles Times* article in July 2009. So, we'll see how it goes.

But enough of that. Would you like some cheese with that whine? On a humorous note, my daughter nearly yanked off my wiener one night. We'd just started using a lift with a sling which hydraulically lifts me out of the chair and over the bed. There was no caregiver on Christmas night, and my wife and daughter were doing fine until I was in bed. Unfortunately for me, the leg strap was wrapped around my urinary catheter tube and firmly attached to my pecker with some adhesive and an elastic Velcro strap around the base. That's when Carey gave a tug on the sling to pull it out from under me. Jeez, Louise! It didn't help that they were both laughing their heads off about her *yankie on the wankie.*

Then one day in January, we planned to see a movie, knowing I could chill the next day. After eating breakfast, I decided it would be more fun to have another sudden attack of explosive diarrhea. We barely made it to the commode chair in the bathroom, and I emptied out so much that I nearly fainted. We turned on the fan, so there is now a new hole in the ozone layer over Camino, California. Jessica still had to use a half can of deodorizer. Anyway, that wiped me out for the week.

On a happier note, I dressed up as Zorro on Halloween (in a black hat, a mask, a cape, and even a whip) and scared the living shit out of some three to four-year-olds who had the door opened by my accomplice. This scary apparition came charging at the front door in a wheelchair with a computer voice saying, "I am Zorro, better watch out for my whip!"

The teenagers thought it was cool and came in the house for photos with me. And I heard one of them say, "Look, he's like Stephen Hawking!" Send that kid off to Harvard.

We hosted an afternoon holiday open house in early December outstandingly catered by our good friend Mike Pingree (his business is called "A Bountiful Cuisine"). I was thinking twenty or thirty people, but Maureen invited about eighty, and sixty-five came. I took an early nap, drank coffee, and took an extra Ritalin (speed), so I got through it. With help from my preprogrammed talking computer, I asked my friends things like, "Who invited you?" and "How's alcohol rehab going? There's beer, wine, and eighteen-year-old scotch in the kitchen." I crashed for two or three days after that party and haven't had the same energy since. But that's okay—go out on a high note and leave 'em laughing.

The PBS documentary that I'm in should air sometime next fall. The website is www.considertheconversation.com. I encourage you to visit the website and donate *generously*, of course.

At Christmas, I sat in my wheelchair surrounded by my wife, children, and my new three-month-old granddaughter Alexis. I felt a warm glow come over me that I will carry to the end. A few days later, we hosted a gathering for my many siblings and their children—another houseful. We have a great photo of us in the living room. All in all, it was a very high and happy note to end the Christmas season.

So that's my story, and I'm sticking to it—who knows what good or ill tomorrow may bring. As a wise man said, "Well, you never know."

THIRTY-FOUR

Fred Tries to Kill Me

~

I lied about having an "ALS Update" in April 2010. By now, you should be used to that. April is over, and it's almost the end of May. Last month was quite a blur, which I'll explain later—and well, I am a congenital liar. So sue me.

We did go to UCSF on April 7. I'd lost about ten pounds, my FVC breathing score had plummeted from 60 percent to 30, and my functional score took a nosedive. We said our goodbyes and sincere thank yous and made the ten-hour trip, which consisted of fifteen minutes with the doc, fifteen minutes with the respiratory therapist, and four tries with four different readings on their wheelchair scale. We weren't at all sure we'd be coming back.

With the "shitty first draft" (to quote author Anne Lamott) of my book done, I mustered a 150 percent effort to look good for all to see at my granddaughter's baptism party. I was following my plan for wrapping things up before my exit, stage left.

I'd been in a wheelchair for two years and was limited to eating pureed food only and drinking only thickened liquids. Even so, I was coughing every time I ate or tried to drink since things were going down the wrong pipe. I hardly ever left the house. Because I was so weak that I could barely stand up, I used bars for transfers. My caregivers were planning how to change my clothes in bed and bring me in the Hoyer Lift over the toilet when I needed to take a crap. And most importantly to me, I was losing dexterity in my hands. That meant I would soon be unable to type, use the talking computer, or drive myself in the wheelchair. Zero quality of life was fast approaching.

I mentally prepared to shut down and stop fighting the pain, frustration, and fear of what was to come—total paralysis. I cut back on eating because I was losing my appetite. I stopped trying to be physically and mentally strong. I became passive, letting others *do* for me instead. And I signed up for hospice on my mother's birthday, March 17, Saint Patrick's Day.

But, nooooooooooooooooo. Instead, I woke up Fred. Now Fred is a mean S.O.B. gnome who lives in your epigastrium (the pit of your stomach). He has a scruffy red beard like an overused Brillo pad, a pipe, and a nasty disposition. Must be Scottish. Fortunately, he mostly sleeps. Occasionally, you catch a glimpse of him in college, after a night of too many margaritas made with cheap tequila. You remember waking up hourly through the early morning, worshiping the toilet, wishing you would die, and soon. But that's just him snorting and turning in his bed.

As a doctor, I can tell you that Fred really wakes up when you have a perforated ulcer or a small stone completely blocking the flow of bile from your gallbladder. He has a nasty brother who lives in your kidneys, but this is not a fricking medical textbook.

Anyway, I don't mean the occasional minor indigestion that people tolerate for a few weeks or months, then schedule *scope* surgery in three weeks on a Friday, so they can start their Hawaiian vacation on Monday. When Fred wakes up, he doesn't screw around. A few of you know what I mean.

Shortly after we started with hospice, Fred decided to wake up one midnight and decided it would be fun to drive a red-hot poker into my midsection to wake me up. Now picture this: I can't talk, am heavily drugged on muscle relaxers and some morphine for the night, and on my BiPAP breathing machine. Maureen is watching TV in the living room (with the baby monitor on, of course, to hear me). Oh, and my legs are paralyzed, it's also pitch dark, and I have trouble calling her since it's agony to move my hands. Soon after this episode, I received an email from someone mentioning my little gallbladder problem, which reminded me of the line from Shakespeare's Romeo and Juliet (Act 2, Scene 2)—"He jests at scars that never felt a wound."

Like any self-respecting doctor, I misdiagnosed myself. I thought I had an ulcer. The pain was *only* in the pit of my stomach, and I figured the stress of it all, blah, blah, blah. When I finally got Maureen in there, she astutely observed that I could hardly breathe from the pain. She gave me the antacid I asked for (thank God for hospice's emergency pack), some more morphine, and a sedative under the tongue. Fred went back to sleep after fifteen minutes, and so did I.

Well, he slept the next night or two, then woke me up in the same evil manner, the pain progressively worsening every few nights. We kept calling hospice in the middle of the night, and they kept saying, "Take more morphine and sedatives." Until I, the brilliant doctor that I am, realized this problem was not the ALS. I decided to have Maureen call 911 for an ambulance at oh-dark-thirty and go to the E.R. for pain relief, mainly because I didn't have a pistol handy to kill myself.

In the E.R., they initially suspected my gallbladder, although the ultrasound wasn't definitive. At least they finally loaded me up on enough narcotics to knock me out (the particular one they chose worked okay, but made me hallucinate like I was on a bad acid trip for the next four days). I'm relying on others for this analogy. I never took acid when I was in college, although as I said earlier, I did smoke a little weed. But again, I digress.

Apparently, the next day, I had a secondary test (which was positive) and surgery that evening. My gallbladder was full of stones and so far gone, it was necrotic (meaning it was about to burst and send awful poisons throughout my abdomen and painfully kill me). Or worse, make me stay in the hospital longer.

Maureen told me later that she was impressed by the mental clarity I'd shown through the pain/haze of a narcotic. It was a great comfort to have the direction from my lips—especially when it was time to make certain decisions: when to go to the E.R. or sign my "X" for surgery. At one point, I told her, "Give me three days." This meant how long to leave the ventilator plugged in if my lungs were too weak after the operation, which is a significant risk with advanced ALS. But it was only fair—Maureen never, ever left me by myself while I was in the hospital. She was either there herself or had arranged for my personal caregivers to be there twenty-four hours a day. After four days of misery and hallucinations, I made it through the crazy experience and we went home.

All was fine until Fred decided that I hadn't had enough yet, so he woke me up again one night maybe two weeks later. It turned out that my liver had a tiny stone stuck in the upper area. Apparently, it had blocked the remaining plumbing on its way back down. Fortunately, I knew what it was and went back to the hospital (another 911 call and an ambulance trip since I was in too much pain to handle the wheelchair—blame me for the Medicare bankruptcy). I spent another two nights in the hospital since the procedure (ERCP) called for general anesthesia. The stay was a relative cakewalk. My personal Fred is now permanently gone, the bastard. May he not rest in peace.

Of course, the saga continued a few weeks later when again, for several nights, I had problems. (Why always at night?) I had some minor chest pains and trouble breathing. One morning, I woke up and my breathing rate was twenty-five times a minute (normal is twelve to twenty), and my pulse was 130 (normal rate is sixty to one hundred). Fortunately, I wasn't in such bad shape that we had to call an ambulance. Maureen drove me to the hospital, so I could sit in my comfortable wheelchair and communicate with my talking computer.

To no one's surprise, I had an extensive array of blood clots in both lungs. The medical schools can use my x-ray and CAT scan as a teaching aid. Fortunately, I stabilized with some supplemental oxygen. The normal treatment for this is a week to ten days in the hospital on an intravenous blood thinner called Heparin. Meanwhile, they gave me a pill called Warfarin which took a while to achieve the same effect of thinning my blood to prevent more clots. Luckily, I could take it orally at home as long as indicated. In my case, it's lifelong.

In my typical fashion, I refused to stay the week to ten days, so we compromised on a different intravenous blood thinner than Heparin called Lovenox (injected under the skin of my belly) and a two-day stay. Of course, this drug is not FDA-approved for treating blood clots in your lungs, but I was a difficult, ornery patient. The home care nurses could come out and give me the shots or teach my caregivers the procedure until the Warfarin was in range. I got my way (I usually do).

Meanwhile, some interesting improvements started happening with my ALS after the gallbladder incident. I was measurably better in several ways that have nothing to do with bile, the gallbladder, or the liver. I won't bore you with all of it, but I started to talk a little again, mostly in the mornings. Breathing and swallowing were also better. Unbelievably, I'm still flexible and take fewer muscle relaxers than months ago. I have strength and coordination in my upper arms that I had lost. My stamina is much better, and I need fewer naps. Neither my doctors nor I have any explanation for this turn of events.

Don't get me wrong; I think ALS is still going to get me. We don't have a miracle cure going here. But at this point, it's nice to have the clock turned back four to six months at least. All of this has given me a new attitude, so I signed off hospice.

Since that time, I've been extraordinarily busy with medical appointments and catching up with family, friends, and emails (the backlog from when I was in a fog). I've also been trying to get my book reorganized and readable, based on the feedback I've received from the agent (who turned down the "shitty first draft") and my personal editors. I have several other good agent contacts and a publisher just waiting to see it. I don't even have time to read and forward funny emails like I used to. I've even done things that weren't possible for the last two years, but I have to stop writing new chapters and work on getting this book ready to publish.

I'm incredibly thankful to those who pulled me through the ordeals described in this chapter, starting, of course, with Maureen. I couldn't have made it without her. Through the haze, I vaguely recall the faces of my daughter, brother, and sisters who visited. And let's not forget the team of caregivers who all chipped in: Jessica, Maria, Leah, Tammy, and Tarah. And somehow, by going through this, I've become spiritually renewed in ways I never imagined. I won't go into details—except to say they involve dead cats and opossum blood under a full moon at midnight. And weird costumes.

Seriously though, I wake up most mornings thankful to be alive, grateful for what I have, and blessed to be surrounded by people who love me. And I spend a few minutes thinking about what all this means. I haven't yet signed on again with hospice; I'm too busy living. I don't think about dying. I think about what I will do today, tomorrow, next week, and in the next few months. It's amazing to me!

Most days, I'm renewed, spoiled rotten, and therefore, happy. I quit antidepressant meds a while ago—that was a no-brainer. Maureen is obviously happier, too. Life is full of surprises. Watch for the good ones that happen to you. They are out there if you pay attention.

As a wise man once said about good news and bad news, "Well, you never know."

APPENDIX A

Remembering Marty

~

The following vignette of Marty is based on an obituary that appeared in the (Placerville, California) Mountain Democrat *on November 4, 2010.*

On October 28, 2010, the community of Placerville lost a unique and special man, Dr. Martin Frederick Welsh, who passed away at the age of fifty-six at his Camino home surrounded by his family. This gentle man's remarkable spirit will be sorely missed.

Martin F. Welsh, M.D., was born in Los Angeles on March 20, 1954, the eldest of six children. He excelled in school—where he loved sports, music, math, and science—and was an inspiration to his younger siblings. Even at a young age he knew that he wanted to be a doctor, an aspiration that spurred him to become the valedictorian of his high school class and then to graduate from UCLA magnum cum laude.

In 1980, Martin graduated from UCLA Medical School and completed his residency at the Ventura County Family Practice Program, where as chief resident, he was known for his keen intellect, wicked sense of humor, and ability to quickly create order out of chaos. In 1983, Martin's dream of becoming a small town family doctor supporting the health of generations of families became a reality when he moved, with his wife Devin and two small children, Carey and Kevin, to Placerville, California, where he established a family medical practice. As a family doctor he was brilliant, energetic, and passionate, even making house calls to patients unable to visit his office.

Martin was a tireless supporter of Marshall Hospital. In 1990, he served as chief of staff, and from 1985 to 1994, he was a member of the

Marshall Hospital Foundation. He was known for his commitment to quality, he served as chair of committees on quality improvement and diabetes care. Martin was the director of the Cameron Park office of Marshall Center for Primary Care. He also continued teaching by serving as assistant clinical professor at the University of California, Davis, Family Practice Program. His reputation as a disciplined and skillful doctor made him sought after as a teacher by student doctors and nurse practitioners. In addition he participated in a variety of other activities linked to his love of sports and music, including coaching his children's basketball team, playing in a basketball league, starting his own rock 'n' roll band called Therapy, and producing a CD entitled *A Little Therapy*. In 2002, he married a second time, to Maureen Gill.

In 2004, Martin was then diagnosed with amyotrophic lateral sclerosis, Lou Gehrig's disease. But despite being challenged by this fatal disease, he maintained a "damn the torpedoes" attitude, practicing medicine as long as his disease allowed and even volunteering with the Flying Samaritans on trips to provide medical services to the poor in San Quintin, Mexico. He also traveled extensively with his wife and joined Cameron Park Country Club, where he played golf until unable to stand on the tee box. Once retired, he wrote, traveled, and inspired others with his passion for life, wacky sense of humor, and remarkable candor about his impending death. He helped raise funds and awareness at many annual walks on behalf of the ALS Association under the banner "Marty's Marchers."

In his final years, Martin's story gained much media attention. He wrote an essay for the *Los Angeles Times* about his end-of-life choices, entitled "Meaning of Life," which was later republished as "100 Things Leading to a Single Choice" in dozens of newspapers throughout the country. His uplifting philosophy about bravely facing the end of life also prompted a filmmaker to feature him in a film about death and dying, the upcoming PBS documentary *Consider the Conversation*.

Martin is survived by his wife Maureen; his children Carey and Kevin; his daughter-in-law Kristen; his granddaughter Alexis; and his five siblings, Katie, Melinda, Tony, Greg, and David.

Life for Marty's children has carried on in many happy and busy ways. His daughter Carey lives in Southern California with her husband Odeh Haddad and their one-year-old son Jackson Martin Hadad. His son Kevin and wife Kristen live in Colorado and have expanded their family. Lexi, now seven years old, has three sisters—Brooke and Edyn (five-year-old twins), and Cora, age three. Marty is missed and always remembered.

For more information about Marty, visit this website.
www.laughtodeathmyrx.com

APPENDIX B

The ALS Rules

~

1. Don't always follow the rules.
2. Know that ALS doesn't always follow its own rules.
3. Remember that I am not the only one who has my ALS.
4. Focus on what I can do, not what I can't do.
5. Have an agenda for every day.
6. Pace myself (and Maureen).
7. Find ways to laugh as much as possible.
8. Have contact every day with family or friends.
9. Focus on and spend time with positive people and things.
10. Contemplating courage for the rest of my life is overwhelming, but courage for today is possible.

Resources

~

The ALS Association
www.alsa.org

This national non-profit organization is at the forefront of the global research effort to find treatments and a cure for ALS. In addition to research, their mission is to serve, empower, and advocate for people affected by ALS to live their lives to the fullest.

The ALS Association Greater Sacramento Chapter
www.alssac.org

The ALS Association Greater Sacramento Chapter supports all people living with ALS, their loved ones, and caregivers with comprehensive support and resources in twenty-four counties throughout California. All of the care services are free of charge and 100 percent funded solely through Chapter fundraising efforts.

Consider the Conversation
www.considertheconversation.org

This film series inspires dialogue about end-of-life issues. *Consider the Conversation* has been broadcast over 2,000 times on PBS stations and garnered twenty-two awards and an Emmy nomination. The first film in the series features Martin F. Welsh, M.D. Purchase the DVD on Amazon.

Foundation for Art and Healing
www.artandhealing.org

Bridging science and the arts, this organization explores the relationship between health and creative expression. They offer innovative programs and tools that empower individuals and engage the community through stories of "art and healing." The UnLonely Project shows how creative expression can help address loneliness in a number of ways.

***Laugh to Death* Website**
www.laughtodeathmyrx.com

Learn more about Martin Welsh and his community. Share your comments and personal stories on the blog. Purchase the book here. Per Martin's wishes, 20 percent of the book sale profits go to The ALS Association Greater Sacramento Chapter.

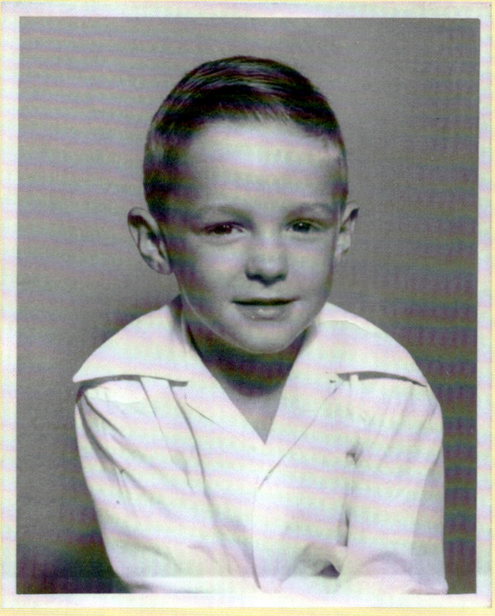

Young Marty, circa late 1950s

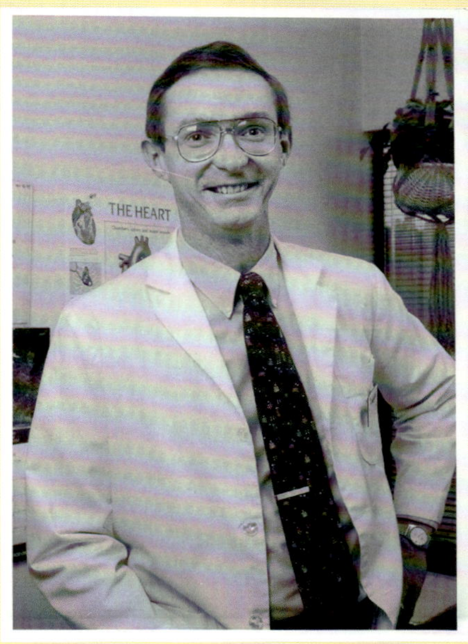

Young Doctor Marty, 1980s

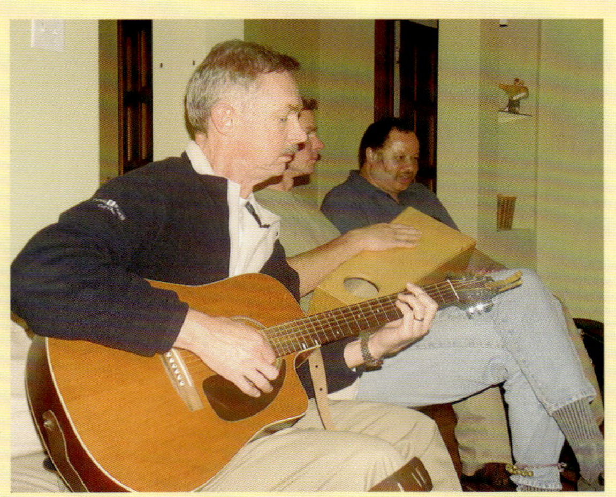

Marty playing guitar at family gathering, 2004

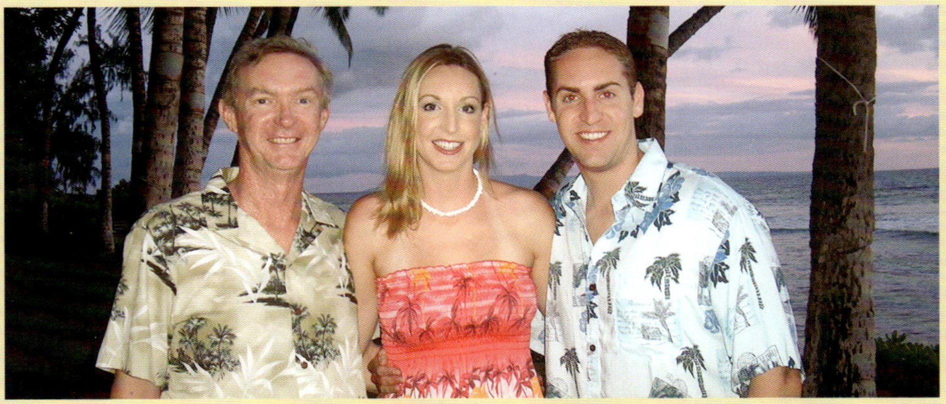

Marty with Carey and Kevin (his kids) in Hawaii, 2005

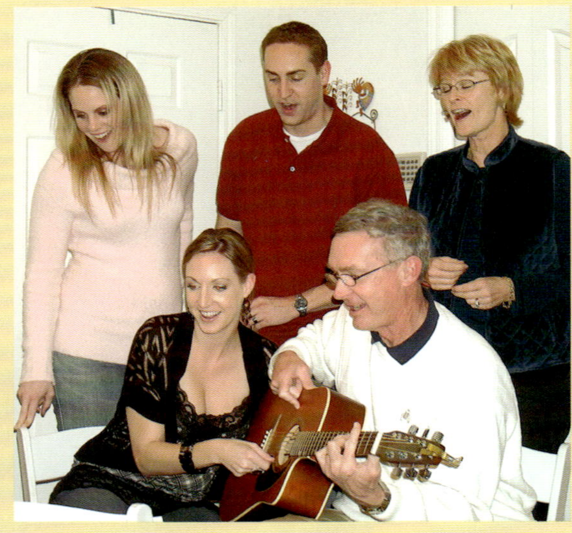

Marty playing guitar at Christmas family gathering, 2006

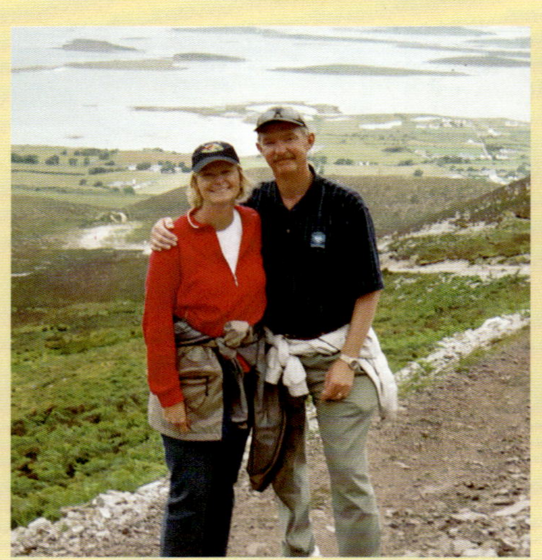

Maureen and Marty hiking up Croagh Patrick Mountain, 2005

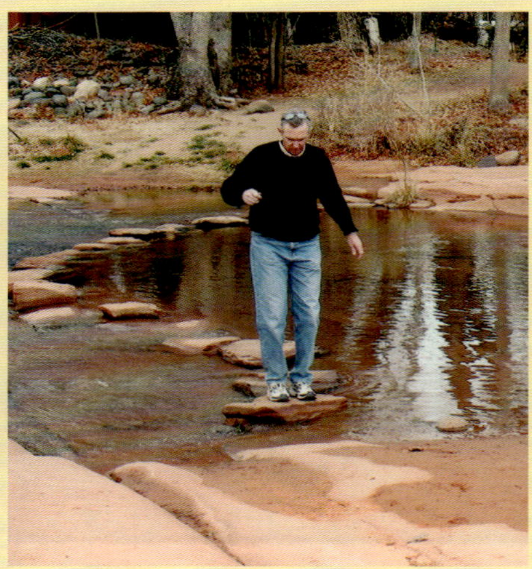

Marty crossing Sedona river, 2006

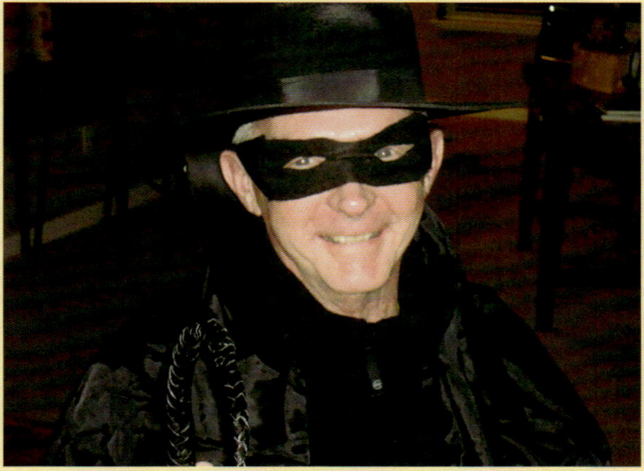

Marty as Zorro on Halloween, 2009

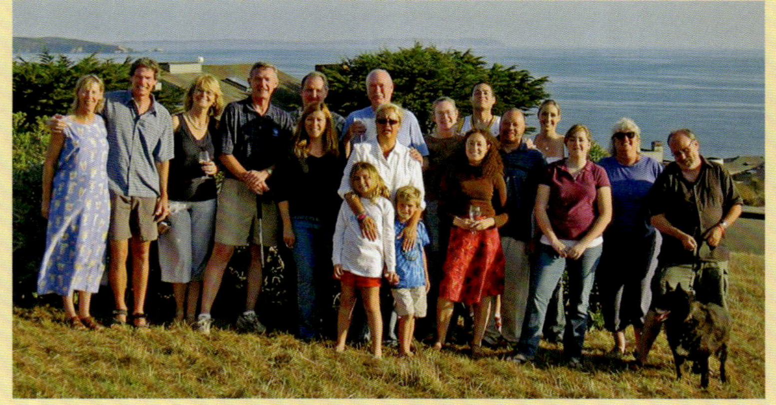

Family gathering at Bodega Bay, 2006

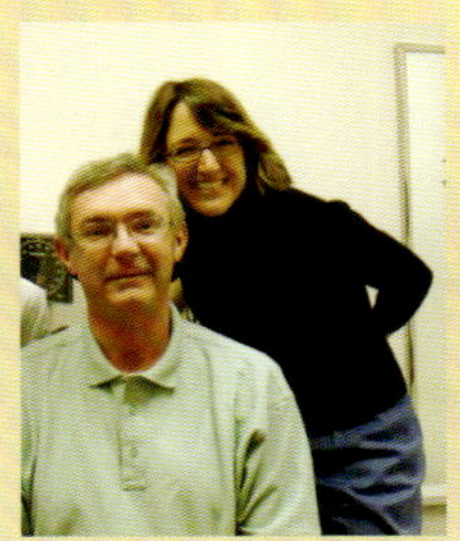

Marty and Dr. Cathy at UCSF, 2008

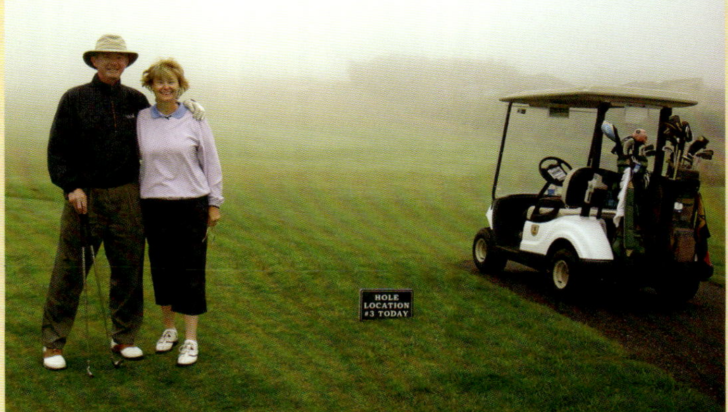

Marty and Maureen golfing at Bodega Bay, 2007

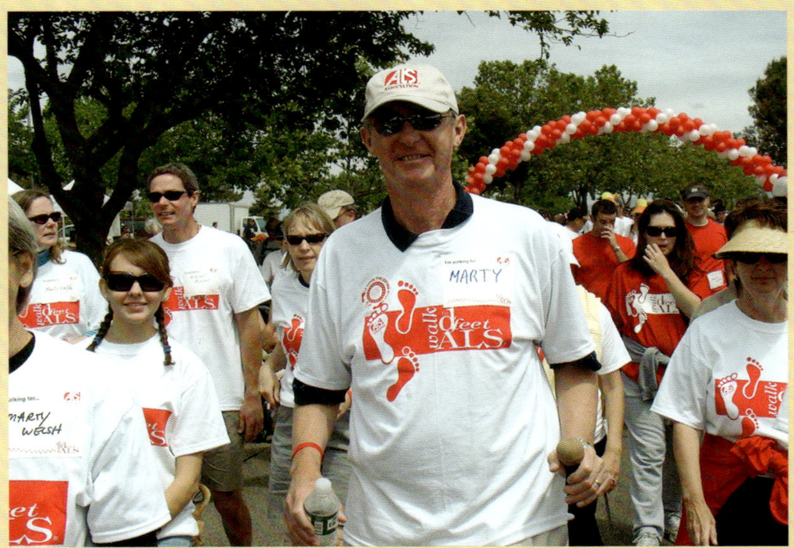

ALS walk, Napa, 2006

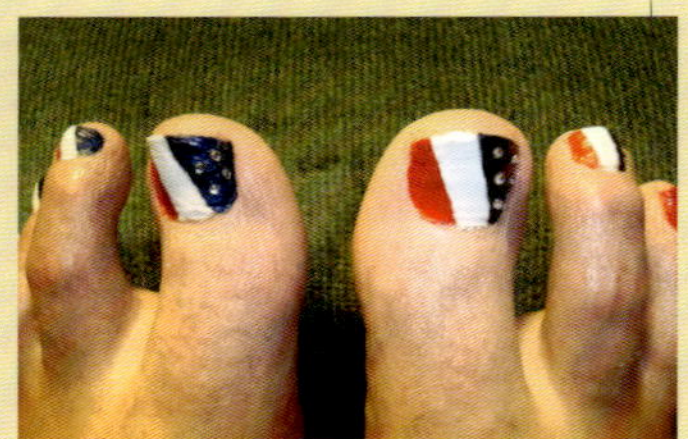

Marty's toes, 2010

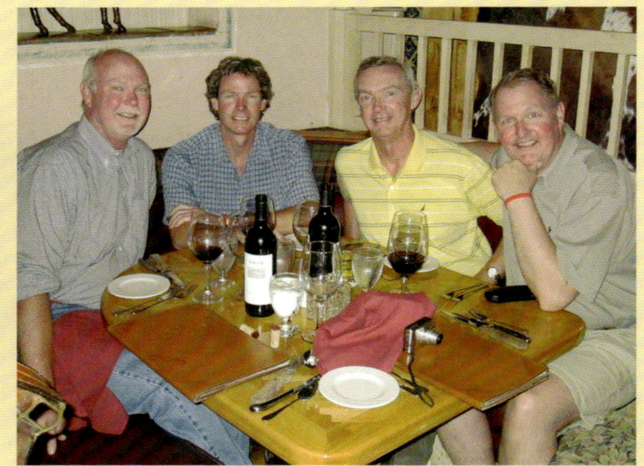

Brothers' weekend fun
Tony, David, Marty, Greg, 2007

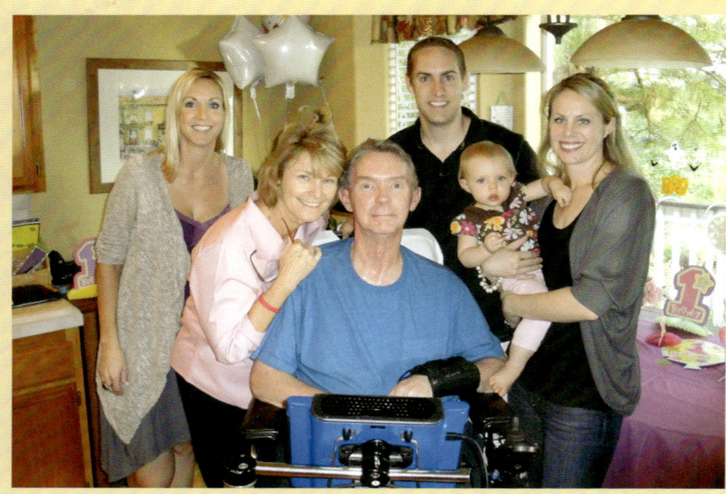

Lexi's first birthday party, 2010

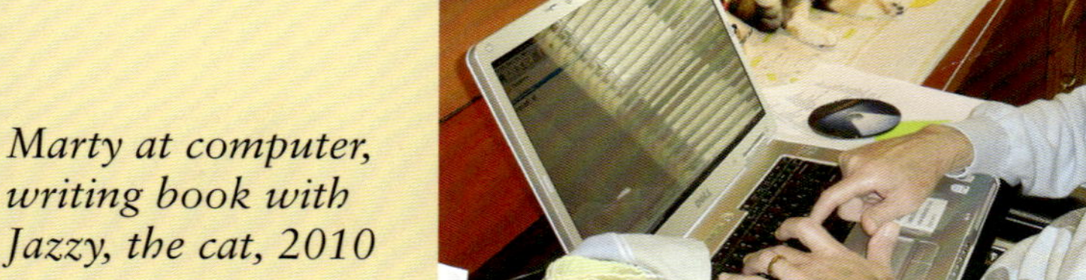

Marty at computer, writing book with Jazzy, the cat, 2010